T0128274

FEED YOURSELF

Fabulous

ASHLEY SIEDENTOPF

BALBOA.PRESS

A DIVISION OF HAY HOUSE

Photographer: Sophie Webster

Balboa Press books may be ordered through booksellers or by contacting:

Balboa Press
A Division of Hay House
1663 Liberty Drive
Bloomington, IN 47403
www.balboapress.com
1 (877) 407-4847

Because of the dynamic nature of the Internet, any web addresses or links contained in this book may have changed since publication and may no longer be valid. The views expressed in this work are solely those of the author and do not necessarily reflect the views of the publisher, and the publisher hereby disclaims any responsibility for them.

The author of this book does not dispense medical advice or prescribe the use of any technique as a form of treatment for physical, emotional, or medical problems without the advice of a physician, either directly or indirectly. The intent of the author is only to offer information of a general nature to help you in your quest for emotional and spiritual well-being. In the event you use any of the information in this book for yourself, which is your constitutional right, the author and the publisher assume no responsibility for your actions.

Any people depicted in stock imagery provided by Getty Images are models, and such images are being used for illustrative purposes only.
Certain stock imagery © Getty Images.

Print information available on the last page.

ISBN: 978-1-9822-3792-9 (sc)
ISBN: 978-1-9822-3794-3 (hc)
ISBN: 978-1-9822-3793-6 (e)

Library of Congress Control Number: 2019917410

Balboa Press rev. date: 05/22/2020

CONTENTS

Feed Yourself Fabulous

A holistic health and nutrition guide to boost your wellbeing, beauty and vitality from within.

- Learn to nourish yourself naturally through nutrition, positive vibes, self-love, and mindfulness.

Fabulous;
amazing, wonderful

F.A.B. (acronym)
stands for fabulous, amazing, beautiful

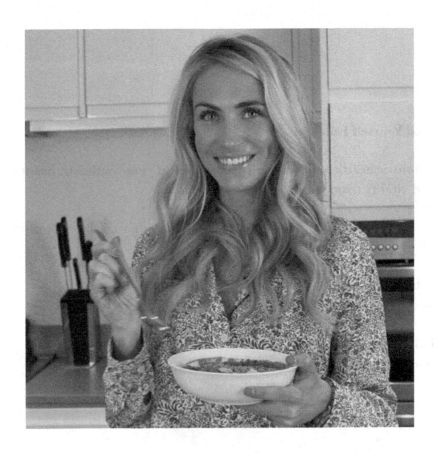

Be your own hero

INTRODUCTION

My book, "Feed Yourself Fabulous," actually had its own little setbacks. Initially, my idea was to create a cookbook; however, I soon realized that what I really wanted was to inspire and make a positive difference for others with my holistic, inside-out approach.

So, I decided to implement the basic wellness tips that I use for my own physical, mental, emotional, and spiritual health; however, after a frustrating mishap with my hard drive, I had to start all over in the summer of 2017. After that, I had a miscarriage, and it left me in a bit of a funk for a few months. I just wasn't feeling like my usually sunny and energetic self. I found out I was pregnant again right before Christmas, and then experienced the suicide of immediate family on my husbands side right after.

Needless to say, experiencing grief during my first trimester depleted my energy on all levels and I tried my best to avoid stress so that I wouldn't have another miscarriage. All in all, I was putting a lot of pressure on myself. Why wasn't my book out already? Why wasn't it done? I felt so bad.

Despite these experiences, or perhaps because of them, my inward journey over this past year and a half was filled with so much growth in all areas of my life, allowing me to refine, add, delete, and polish my story and work along the way.

In hindsight, I supposed it worked out better this way, because I get to share some of the wisdom that I've learned through my setbacks. To be honest, as cliché as it sounds, those times of struggle or sadness truly make you stronger, wiser, and better if you allow yourself to accept, let go, and learn from it.

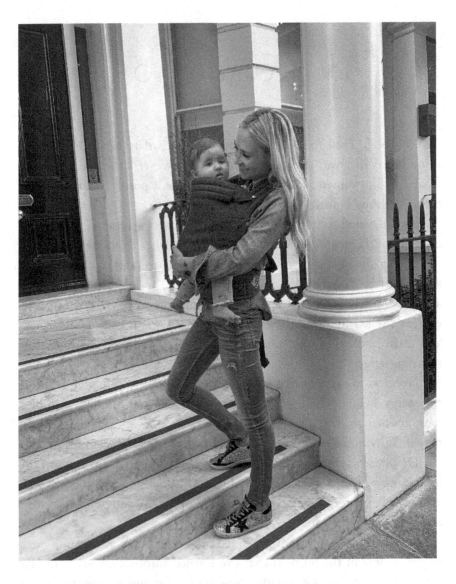

Have courage, be kind, stay humble and love life

MY STORY

No one enjoys enduring the hardships of life, but sometimes, they help us find a greater purpose. Such was the case for me. My personal experience with medical hardship and my desire to learn about the importance of a whole-food-based diet are what led me down the path of studying nutrition.

It all started when I was 11 years old. I experienced some pretty painful, inexplicable symptoms regularly for over a year. On my twelfth birthday, in March of 1995, I was finally diagnosed with Crohn's Disease. I remember lying in a hospital bed with an IV drip, completely shocked, terrified, and speechless.

They pumped my body full of high-dose steroids in an attempt to reduce inflammation. The doctors ultimately had no answers as to what happened or why. The only pain relief that worked was Demerol and Morphine — a narcotic drug used to treat moderate to severe pain and comes with serious side effects including nausea and dizziness.

The most horrific part of those 10 days in the hospital were the tests and examinations. I was poked several times, was given an endoscopy, colonoscopy, MRI, and a Barium Swallow, where I had to drink 2–3 litres of a vile, chalky liquid. These procedures became part of my life.

After I was released, I was prescribed Cortisone, which is a steroid that prevents the release of substances in the body that cause inflammation. This caused my face to swell, and it gave me mood swings, sweats, insomnia, and a very large appetite. I was also given Pentasa, a drug that was supposed to heal my gut but worsened the symptoms my hair started falling out, I felt sick after eating, and I experienced severe headaches.

Over the years, I was in and out of hospitals, tube-fed, and put on medication after medication. I was missing a lot of school and falling behind, so my parents decided to switch things up and try a holistic approach.

When I was 14, I had my first consultation with the Naturopathic Doctor. He gave me a long list of foods to avoid that seemed daunting, and the number of supplements he prescribed me seemed scary: digestive enzymes, fish oils, Vitamin B and D shots, L-Glutamine, Ester C, Probiotics, etc.

Within a few months, I had no stomach aches, no toilet troubles, and my appetite was back to normal again. I was absolutely thrilled — and my doctors were surprised too. They had never mentioned *anything* about **ditching dairy, sugar, wheat, gluten, and other processed-type foods.**

However, as time went on and I approached my early twenties, my health started to decline again due to poor eating habits and lifestyle choices. **Flare-ups were worse, the pain was excruciating, and hospital visits became longer.**

At the age of 23, I was living in Athens for the summer, and my condition was so brutal that I visited the hospital. The doctors said it could have been fatal if I had not come to the hospital that day.

The tests had revealed a large stomach abscess. Bacteria had entered my body, and my immune system was trying to fight the infection by sending white blood cells to the infected area. As the white blood cells attacked the bacteria, it caused inflammation, pain, and the death of nearby tissue, leading to the formation of a cavity.

Being bed-bound for two weeks in a foreign hospital with very poor conditions around me led to a profound moment of truth and acceptance: I have a disease, and the only one who can help me is ME.

I am still an extremely sensitive and delicate person today, not just emotionally, but health-wise too. Through managing Crohn's to hypothyroidism, food allergies, and asthma, I HAVE to put my health first. If I don't, or if I'm too stressed or make poor nutrition and lifestyle choices, I experience tummy troubles, breathing problems, lethargy, insomnia, anxiety, skin rashes — you name it. Call me "Sensitive Suzy."

One thing I know for sure is that your mind is the most powerful tool you have. I never let the disease define me. Every time I have been hit with a painful, debilitating flare-up, I am reminded to have faith, stay positive, pray, and not submit to being a victim of an illness.

When I was stuck in that hospital bed in Athens, I decided to take personal responsibility for my health. I took charge. I made a tremendously empowering commitment to myself that I would try my best to never be in that situation again.

Since then, I've found my passion and insatiable appetite for learning about health and nutrition — not only for myself, but also for my friends, family, and everyone I care about. I will always have to live with an autoimmune disease, but that doesn't mean it defines me; it only makes up a small part of me, and I don't let it take over my life. I listen to my body, and if I am feeling unwell, fatigued, or just generally not full of energy, I slow down with lots of self-care. I take a time-out, and I try to add more nourishing foods, thoughts, and holistic therapies to my routine, including acupuncture, reiki, and massages for extra healing.

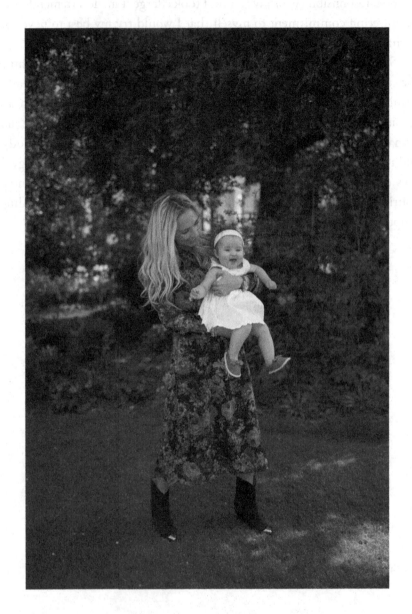

I am always with you, be happy, be humble,
be kind, have courage and love life

ME IN A NUTSHELL

I'm Ashley. I am a certified nutritionist and integrative nutrition health coach, wellness enthusiast, health and beauty writer, cooking and health talk host, skincare creator, wifey, mama, pug mama, and lover of food, fashion, sunshine, photography, travelling, yoga, pilates, reading, wine, cooking, and spending time with loved ones. I am a free-spirit, life-loving, doesn't-take-herself-too-seriously kind of chick.

Today at 36, I have conquered Crohn's disease, lived in six different countries, and have worked in all trades from front of house, to fashion, eventually finding my true passion for food. I don't just mean the stuff you eat on your plate — I am talking about **the nourishing foods for your mind, body, soul, and spirit.**

By definition, *fabulous* means, "amazing, wonderful." For me, **fabulous is living your life fully**. It's eating an abundance of nutritious, natural foods. It's choosing work that makes you want to jump out of bed — work that brings you joy. It's dressing up and looking your best, no matter what your budget is. It's tapping in spiritually to awaken and unlock your true potential. It's being in love with YOU, moving daily, and just simply feeding yourself fabulous, from nourishing mantras and mat workouts to delicious, healthy meals — all to become F.A.B. (i.e. fabulous, amazing, beautiful — you'll see this used throughout this book).

I want to share with other women how you can eat, feel, live, and look fab from the inside out. But don't get me wrong: I didn't wake up one day and decide to become fabulous.

Rather, my knowledge, studies, and focus, as well as my life experiences — big breakups, financial troubles, a nearly fatal experience in Athens that left me bedridden, bereavement of loved ones from both sickness and suicide, and living with an autoimmune condition better known as Crohns disesase— have hugely influenced who I am today as a person.

I now look at life through a different lens. I have chosen to never waste a moment on NOT living my life to the fullest and most fabulous, simply appreciating the gift of life has to offer and the privilege of being. After realising we are only on Earth for a limited amount of time, I try to live, love, laugh, and enjoy life every day.

What I've come to realize is that both good and bad experiences are connected in a beneficial way. Passions, special gifts, talents, education, background, personality, purpose, imperfections, and setbacks — shape who we are. For me, it's being an advocate for positive thinking, embracing the best parts of me, having a grateful heart, eating healthy, practicing mindfulness, living fully, moving daily, nurturing close connections, being compassionate towards myself, and living a high vibe lifestyle. The more I adopted this holistic approach to life, the more I've started to live life in the fab lane.

Life can be full of great surprises, struggles, and setbacks, but no matter what your background and life story is, it is up to you how you feel, eat, live, and look — no pill, potion, or person is going to help you feel and look fab except you.

Learning to accept and love who you are, living life to the fullest, and focusing on things that make you happy and joyful will turbo-boost your mind, body, soul, and spirit into fabulosity.

I am an advocate for an integrative approach to optimizing health & wellness through meditation. I also encourage the practice of mindfulness, intuitive eating, uplifting affirmations, mantras, movement, gratitude, and a whole lot of self-love, all of which will be broken into small fragments throughout the book. I am a firm believer that when you feel well from nourishing meals, boost your endorphins from daily movement, and have a positive, happy mindset, you will be able to stay on the path of growth, love, peace, joy, abundance, and beauty to live your best possible life.

After graduating from nutrition school, I launched ashfab.net, an online destination for natural health information, nutrition, fitness, beauty, and wellness tips, as well as programs, product reviews, cooking videos and interviews with fellow fabulous females. This website reflects my philosophy: Nutrition for natural beauty from the inside out to help you feel and look fab holistically. From nourishing meals to mat workouts and mantras, the combination can truly bring your natural beauty from the inside out.

Beauty is not just about having glowing skin, a strong body, slim waistline, and lustrous hair; rather, a beautiful soul feels, acts, and thinks with love, kindness, and compassion towards herself and others. A beautiful soul is never jealous, judgmental, resentful, or negative toward others' success or "better" lifestyle. Beautiful women accept where and who they are and are happy for others as well. Feeling and looking fabulous comes down to a formula.

Using my background, experience, and studies in health and nutrition, I wanted to channel my enthusiasm toward wellness to inspire fellow females and make a difference to help them become the most F.A.B. versions of themselves through holistic methods like thinking positively, staying present, holding powerful self-beliefs, and choosing a diet dominated by natural nutrition.

It is vital to work on your inside beauty first. The best places to start are feeding your body with an abundance of plant-based foods, staying hydrated, taking supplements so your cells can thrive, followed by nurturing your mind with uplifting affirmations, mantras, meditation, visualizations, positive thinking, prayer (if it suits your beliefs), and a grateful heart.

The next step is learning to live large, think big, surround yourself with nature, beauty, art, and joy, go on new adventures, love yourself fully, and continue your education, all of which will allow you to evolve and grow into the greatest version of yourself.

Finally, it will be time to work on your outside beauty & self-love with daily movement (this will boost your mood and metabolism, and it will melt fat for a healthy and strong body), a daily skin routine, good grooming habits to look polished and put-together, and finding a style to suit your personality that boosts your confidence and makes you feel great.

"Feed Yourself Fabulous" is a holistic approach to upgrading your health, body, beauty, and spirit. It is a holistic lifestyle guide to eating, feeling, living, and looking fab, as well as an easy-to-follow outline of things I do in my life that nourish me naturally from the inside out.

This book shows you how to eat fab, feel fab, live fab and look fab. It is divided into four parts so you can refer back to these tips any time to give you that boost you may need seasonally.

This is not a restrictive, obsessive diet. It is not calorie counting or a quick fix to help you shed pounds. Rather, it is a holistic lifestyle that will encourage you to be the most fab version of yourself from the inside out. After all, why be ordinary when you can be extraordinary?

A holistic approach is a form of healing that considers you as a whole person from the inside out; it's making sure your mind, body, spirit, and emotional health are all in balance. It is listening to that burning desire inside of you that wants change and is constantly seeking optimal health, wellness, and ways to feel and look your best today.

This lifestyle combines a mind-body-spirit style of medicine with mindful thinking, eating, acting, and moving. I want you to be excited about this new path of feeding your body with fabulous food to help you feel and look amazing from the inside out. By eating fabulous foods, you will naturally crowd out the crappy foods that make you feel and look bad. You'll say, "bye-bye!" to bloating, blotchy skin, and brain fog, and "hello!" to lots of energy, glowing skin, and vibrant health. I will help you begin this journey — all I need from you is dedication, discipline and devotion.

Think of it this way: imagine yourself waking up, feeling amazing. You get out of bed, full of enthusiasm toward a new day, feeling joyful, well, and energetic. You find it easy to give your full attention to your family and friends, and when you go to bed, your heart is grateful, and most importantly you love yourself very much (rather than being a judgmental jerk to yourself).

You deserve to live the kind of life that we all dream about. If and when there are setbacks and struggles, choose to look at the bright side as much as possible. Surrender through the obstacles, accept them, let them go, have faith in a brighter future, and stay present. Through life's toughest times, we become wiser, stronger, and more resilient.

Why feel fine when you can feel fabulous? Why look fine when you can look fabulous? Why sell yourself short and live small, when you can be fabulous, exude confidence, and act boldly? Why live fine, just getting through each day, struggling and letting life pass you by, when you can live fabulously? It is so important to have the highest, grandest visions of yourself and your life, so adopt a fabulous mindset TODAY!

Feel it, believe it, and see it — don't wait for the future. Start now! Say to yourself out loud, "I am fabulous, and I am feeding my body from this day forward with only the most nourishing food, thoughts, and movement. I commit to beautifying myself from the inside out." Fabulous meals, mantras, mindfulness, and mat workouts will truly make you feel and look your best!

"A strong, positive, optimistic mindset is paramount to vibrant health."

—Ashley Siedentopf

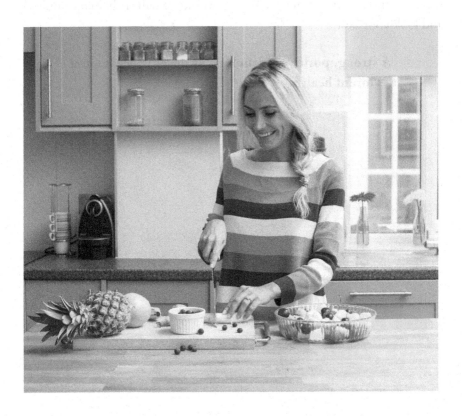

Make meal times an enjoyable thing, savour
the flavour and bless that moment

A LITTLE ABOUT
ME & MY STORY

I was born and raised in Edmonton, Canada, a city of 900,000 people with a small-town feel and four seasons, especially cold winters. My humble beginnings took place here.

I've also lived in L.A., London, Milan, Vancouver, a few places in Greece & the South of France, and I spent my summers from 6-weeks-old until my late teens in the British countryside with my mum's family; these are my Earth roots — they helped shape who I am today.

I believe where I was brought up, and where I have lived up until now, with extensive travel around the world, has opened my eyes, cultivated me, and educated me in a way that no degree or PHD could have. My experiences around the world helped me connect with others on all levels, enabling me to be a chameleon in diverse environments so I could adapt and immerse myself into many different situations.

I was always that little girl who had big dreams, who wanted to live a colorful life. When I was in high school, everyone around me was applying to local universities to study teaching, nursing, or engineering — but none of these subjects really lit my passion. I could not connect with this path in any way, shape, or form.

Instead, I decided to enroll in a selection of classes from different fields such as anthropology, psychology, and political science because I wanted to be able to say I tried and at least gave it a chance. However, this route just didn't give me that feeling of joy. Something felt empty deep inside of me, so I decided to continue on my soul-searching journey. In my early 20s, I left for Vancouver for seven months, and the rest is history.

I am so happy I decided not to follow the path that seemed so normal to others. By the time I was 21 years old, many of my peers had graduated, gotten engaged, bought a condo, and lived a comfy life; however, I thought to myself, "Nope! I have my whole life to settle down and be cushy!`` In 2004, I flew to Milan to study fashion, followed by London in 2005, and I've been Europe-bound ever since.

My upbringing, background, diverse circle of friends, and different fields of work, as well as the amazing teachers, mentors, healers, and hotshots I met along the way taught me a lot about life. When I look back, I think of all the fond memories I have and how they opened my eyes. I remember all that I have overcome and experienced, and everything I've learned from life. Being around different people and places taught me about flexibility, adaptability, and gave me a deep understanding of many scenarios and situations.

So aside from my approach to diet and the importance of natural nutrition, the tips and tools I discuss throughout the book are really an accumulation of all the lessons, inspiration, and wisdom I have learned on my wellness journey throughout the years that work for me and that I want to share with you — sharing is caring, after all:

If you can manage to take away at least one tip from this book that makes a difference in your life, it will mean the world to me and fill my heart with gratitude.

> **"When you merge into different surroundings, meet new people, have new experiences, and step out of your comfort zone, it can change the way you think about yourself and your future in a positive light!"**
>
> **—Unknown**

Imagine yourself as a radiant beauty, strong and healthy, glowing and happy, free from pain and discomfort, full of optimism, joy, gratitude and enthusiasm. This is *absolutely* possible. It's normal to have some bad days — they're just a part of life. However, it is our birthright to be happy and healthy. The only thing you need to do is decide right here, now, that is what you want!

Recently, I questioned my own path and health. Even though my life was going well for the most part, I knew deep down that after my miscarriage, my body had not fully recovered. Despite my doctors insisting that my blood work was normal and healthy, I was very weak and just wasn't feeling "Ash-fab" and full of life. I decided to make healing holistically my priority and to start giving myself extra self-love and self-care.

I booked a session for *Vega testing*, a bioenergetic regulatory technique that measures the body's electrical energy activity through acupuncture points. Vega testing reads cell damage and measures bodily changes due to biologically incompatible substances, such as toxins, bacteria, parasites, heavy metals, etc. I discovered some imbalances that the doctors did not detect caused by the miscarriage, my overworked immune system, and my under-active thyroid. These imbalances were leaving me feeling wiped out all the time.

I started homeopathic remedies made from plants and flowers which worked wonders. I soon began to feel Ashfab again.

I wanted to do everything in my power to optimize my health, recover naturally, rejuvenate my fertility, and heal holistically. I also enrolled in additional therapies to boost my inner and outer health, including reiki, cupping, deep tissue massage sessions, and weekly acupuncture.

Since my 35th birthday was approaching, I decided then and there: I wanted to reach my absolute full potential. I wanted vibrant health, so I committed to feasting on beautifying foods and ditching toxic triggers, only allowing myself to consume unhealthy foods occasionally, and because I discovered imbalances with Vega testing that doctors did not catch with a regular blood test, I decided to go all-in. I know myself better than anyone else — and that is the beauty of paying attention, being mindful, and listening to your body, even if doctors say, "You're OK," when deep down, you know something is just not right.

It is better to do your own research and perhaps book an appointment with a naturopath to discover the root of the problem, as I was misdiagnosed about five different times with Crohn's disease and an under-active thyroid. I've been retested, and my thyroid is perfectly normal now. I was also able to conceive again, which is a huge blessing that I am absolutely over the moon about.

If you are experiencing pain, suffering from tummy troubles, feel tired constantly, can't seem to shift the weight, are not rocking a clear and glowing complexion, or just do not feel amazing, it is time for you to ask yourself questions and do daily body scans.

Of course, life is not always peachy, and you may have days that are not great due to overworking, travel, too many social engagements, or simply indulging too much over the holidays. However, for the most part, it is your birthright to be healthy, feel fantastic, look your best at any age, exude vitality and radiance, and rock that glow factor, whether you're 27 or 77.

My holistic lifestyle guide explains the four pillars of wellness, which is my approach to unleashing vibrant health, well-being, and natural beauty from the inside out. The book is divided into four parts with all my tips, tricks, and tools to help you become the most fabulous version of yourself holistically and to transform your mind, body, beauty, and spirit naturally.

I want you to learn how to eat, feel, live and look your most fabulous. This is no quick fix diet by any means. Instead, it is a long-term lifestyle solution to live fabulously. I promise that after just 10 days of total commitment to this program, you will feel good, look great, and develop habits that will stay with you for life.

If you're not feeling your best, there is hope! Simply follow the included nutritional guidelines, make it a habit to nourish your body with natural nutrition, and implement all the other tips to boost your mental, emotional, and spiritual health.

Life is precious, and we only have one, so let's choose a fabulous mindset! Stay dedicated, disciplined, and devoted to yourself, because you deserve to feel fabulous! As soon as you adopt the fab attitude, your life will begin to feel and look fabulous. By the end of the book, you can use these tips every single day to eat, live, feel, and look better — plus, I have included 30 healthy recipes to help boost, balance, and beautify your body from the inside out.

"Food, fitness and a fabulous mindset is the foundation to feeling and looking great!"

—Ashley Siedentopf

Ashfab Tip: It takes 21 days to adopt a healthy habit, but it takes 66 days to break a bad one. Try committing to a new habit for just THREE days. When you succeed, try it for six, then nine. Before you know it, day 10 will come, and you'll experience a boost in motivation to continue working toward your goals.

If this is a huge change for you, you will probably feel a little worse before you feel better, as your body adjusts to your new lifestyle. Be dedicated, devoted, and disciplined in your personal development and growth, follow the guidelines, and evolve into the beautiful, glowing goddess you deserve to be.

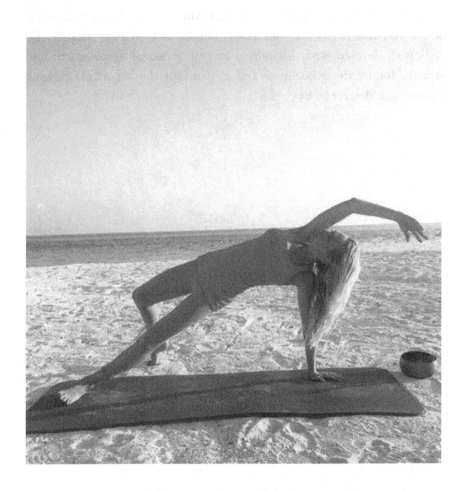

I do yoga to burn off the crazy

Let's do this!

Feed yourself fabulous is divided into four pillars of wellness: Eat Fab, Feel Fab, Live Fab & Look Fab

Eat Fab

The Eat Fab pillar covers the importance of natural nutrition and adding an abundance of plants to your daily diet, as well as tips and tools to help you understand imbalances in your body. This includes meal ideas, seasonal shopping lists, and a beauty-food feasting guide for vibrant health, glowing skin, loads of energy, slim waistline, strong nails, lustrous hair, better mood, memory, and sleep patterns.

This is not a quick fix diet — it's not calorie-counting, deprivation, or rigidity either. It's a guide to having a healthy relationship with food, educating yourself about your health, and choosing fresh, natural ingredients for health-boosting and beautifying benefits.

Feel Fab

The Feel Fab pillar focuses on how to become mindful of your thoughts, feelings, and actions by focusing on healthy, happy, positive vibes, releasing negative self-limitations and talk, learning to love yourself whole-heartedly, and using holistic therapies to boost inner health. The main goal of the Feel Fab pillar is to show you that self-care is the best type of healthcare.

You will learn how to create and maintain balance in your Chakra system by opening, aligning and activating your Chakras. You will learn how to express emotions, journal your thoughts, and do daily mind dumps for instant therapy.

Live Fab

The Live Fab pillar will help you live your best life today! You'll learn how to live fully, be proactive, go after what you want, and manifest your dreams until they happen. You'll cleanse your body and mind of toxic emotions and harmful vibes like fear, doubt, anger, and judgment. And you'll learn to follow your heart — because when you follow the whispers of your soul, you are co-creating a life you love, and this will bring natural happiness to your life.

Look Fab

The Look Fab pillar will help you make daily movement part of your routine so that you can build a strong, healthy body. You will also discover a daily skincare regime to restore radiance and boost brightness. This pillar will teach you the importance of adopting a sense of style to bring out your best features, whether it's bold prints and colors or a more minimalist look with jaw-dropping accessories.

Taking pride in your physical appearance boosts confidence, self-esteem, and self-love, and, by taking care of your appearance, you are also implementing self-care into your lifestyle.

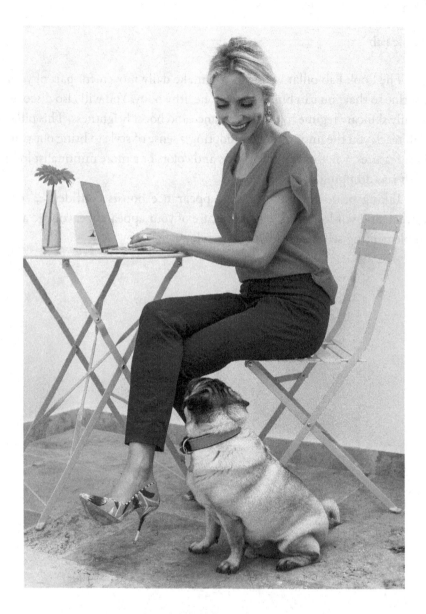

Let your confidence shine, choose courage
because bravery will reward you for it

PART 1

Eat Fab

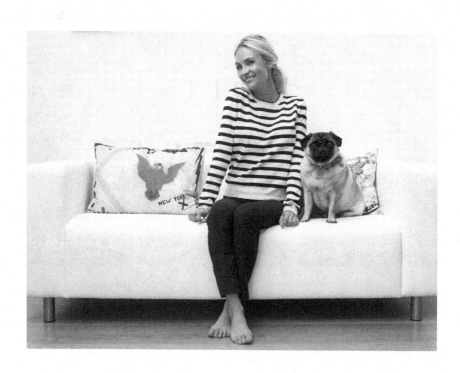

A dog will be your best friend no matter what

Consume foods that make you feel and look fab from the inside out.

In today's day and age, we lead extremely busy lives that leave us little to no time at all for cooking nourishing meals that give us energy and vitality — meals that optimize our overall health and wellness. This chapter shows you how to eat delicious meals that are full of fresh produce, plant protein, texture, and taste that will provide you with the perfect balance of carbohydrates, fats, protein, fiber, minerals, and vitamins.

Healthy food doesn't have to be bland and boring! I love food, so with wholesome ingredients combined with herbs and spices, you get fabified fun food full of vital nutrients to optimize your health. You will find everything from nutrient-rich smoothies to sumptuous soups and simple, savoury suppers.

My recipes and cooking style use ingredients that are fresh, nourishing and simple, so I can prepare meals that are made in minutes. They are the perfect, nutrition-based combination of healthy, varied, and balanced. You'll see that being healthy isn't about rigidness, deprivation, starvation, or calorie-counting. By implementing nutrient-dense foods into your daily life, you'll experience health, wellness, and beauty benefits.

Nutrition plays a vital role in our overall health, wellness, and beauty, so when you give your body real food, it will respond in ways you would never imagine. It is often said "we are what we eat," but it is actually more accurate to say, "we are what we absorb and digest." By choosing an abundance of natural nutrition such as fruit, vegetables, legumes, nuts, seeds, sprouts, sea vegetables, staple starches, gluten-free whole-grains, cold-pressed oils, organic fish, and if you choose to eat animal protein, organic poultry and occasional grass-fed beef, you will start to feel and see a difference in no time.

Most healthy people take personal control of their health. They make mindful choices about what they eat and drink and how they think and act. They know that they are in charge of all habits, good and bad.

By taking personal responsibility for your health and integrating bite-sized healthy habits into your daily life, you will soon realize the power of good nutrition and start to see small changes soon after. I don't want to restrict you to a particular label — I simply want to encourage and inspire you to nourish your body with natural nutrition — so my recipes are dominated by plants. They are energizing, immune-boosting, inflammation-fighting, beautifying, and nutrient-dense (i.e. high in nutrients and low in calories).

As I want to encourage you to nourish your health, well-being, and beauty with predominantly plant-based nutrition, there are over 30 recipes to choose from, all free from refined sugar, cows milk, gluten, and meat.

Simply focus on the beauty food feasting list, instead of focusing on what you can't eat, turn your attention to what you can eat. That way, you will feel empowered by nourishing your health and beauty, and get inspired to get creative in the kitchen. Simply save 2–3 small meals at supper time or spread out over the weekend for your favourite moorish meals.

When you make beauty food feasting part of your lifestyle, you strengthen your immune system, banish bloat, have better digestion, melt fat, gain more energy, have healthier hair, stronger nails, glowing skin, and a clear complexion — overall, you achieve optimal health, which combats accelerated aging and illness.

By following a diet dominated by natural nutrition and abundance of plants, you naturally crowd out C.R.A.P. (Cows milk, Refined foods, Artificial flavors, and Processed foods); furthermore, I find that if you are starting your day right, you will end it right too. After day 10 of completing the program, you will feel amazing and be more mindful of what you put in your mouth. And when you have a "treat day," you'll enjoy every bite as you eat slowly and savor the moment.

I have provided a basic guide of how to eat healthy along with a selection of meal ideas, including over 30 recipes you can use again and again. Most of these recipes require little time, so with proper meal planning, smart shopping, and food prepping, you're on your way to the fab lane.

If you end up stuck or unable to find the time to cook that day, simply research local, organic cafes that offer similar style dishes that are freshly prepared and full of produce.

I wanted to keep this short, sweet, and simple, so instead of giving you 60 recipes, I've chosen my top seven favorites for each category. These recipes are full of flavor, easy to make, and packed with nourishing, beautifying properties — and best of all, I never get tired of them, so you won't either!

As there are millions of books, guides, tips, tricks, and diets related to "healthy eating," **I don't want to overload you with information that leaves you feeling overwhelmed, frazzled, and not-so-motivated** when it comes to food. I'd rather inform and inspire you by sharing my tips, tricks, and tools for vibrant health, glowing skin, a slim waistline, and a positive attitude that will help you on your health and wellness journey.

I am living proof of the benefits that come with beauty food feasting, from healing Crohn's disease naturally, maintaining my healthy weight, and feeling energized and fabulous at 36. That's why I want to share my message with fellow females around the world — I want you to feel the same surge of energy I do, to have vibrant health, to look and feel your best at any age.

Once you reduce the foods that are sabotaging your success and decrease the toxicity, you can achieve weight loss and wellness goals that will last a lifetime. You will also feel and look fabulous in the process.

Remember, it's all about balance. Once you have stuck to the food plan for 10 days, you can allow room for the occasional indulgences. When your body is functioning at an optimal level, your body can handle treats and break it down much better. Balance is key to having a healthy mindset about food.

> **"I stay away from obsessive diets, labels, and calorie counting. Having a flexitarian approach to food leaves no room for deprivation or rigidness when it comes to diet; however, I do feel healthier, happier, and more empowered when I eat nutrient-dense foods that fuel me and heal my body."**
>
> **—Ashley Siedentopf**

Ashfab Fact: Nutrient-dense means high in nutrients and low in not-so-healthy things. By contrast, processed foods are high in empty calories and low in nutrients.

By choosing foods that help you rather than harm you, you will enjoy more energy, improve your digestion, have glowing skin, jumpstart your metabolism, and reduce unwanted belly bloat; not to mention, you'll have a positive mindset and feel more optimistic and enthusiastic about life — when you eat well, your mind and mood are sharper, more focused, and switched on.

Often people find themselves feeling confused about what to eat, and when that happens, they end up eating foods that stress the body instead of fuel it — or worse, they just go hungry, becoming overly rigid and deprived of our favourite things. So keep it simple, fresh, and natural.

> **"Having lived in France, Italy, and Greece, I noticed that food is an important part of life. There's nothing like sitting down for a nice home-cooked meal with loved ones, eating slowly, and enjoying that moment without feeling guilty, or depriving yourself. This is key to having a good relationship with food: use seasonal, fresh, natural ingredients and savor the moment."**
>
> **—Ashley Siedentopf**

Benefits of Natural Nutrition

Boost, balance, & beautify your body from the inside out.

Natural nutrition comes with amazing benefits, such as:

- Strong immune system
- Glowing skin
- Clear complexion
- Strong nails & lustrous hair
- Good digestion
- Better mood & memory
- Less bloat & belly fat
- Slim waistline
- Better sleep
- Ability to fight inflammation

- Less oxidative stress (which accelerates ageing & lifestyle illness)
- Fewer aches & pains
- Loads of energy
- Balanced hormones
- Reduced aging effects

Natural nutrition also reduces your risk of:

- Stroke
- Cardiovascular disease
- Type 2 diabetes
- Obesity
- Heart disease
- Some cancers

If you struggle with the any of following, this may be a sign that your body is deficient in key nutrients & carrying too many toxins:

- Weight gain
- Belly fat
- Asthma
- Joint pain & arthritis
- Back pain
- Skin problems like rashes, pimples, and prominent wrinkles
- Bloating
- Inflammation in the body
- Fatigue & lethargy
- Brain fog
- Cellulite
- Dry lips

Predominantly Plant-Based Nutrition:

Meals that are made from plants with few to no animal products help boost, balance, and beautify your body from the inside out. If you choose to eat animal products in moderation, which I do as well, make sure the animals are raised organically, grass-fed, and locally sourced.

A diet that is dominated by meat, wheat, cow's milk, refined sugar, processed foods, and alcohol is a recipe for inflammation. Inflammation is how your body responds to injury — on the surface, inflammation appears red, hot, painful, and swollen; however, on a cellular level, chronic disease thrives in areas of silent inflammation.

There are many signs of inflammation that you should pay attention to. As you eat more and more plant-based nutrition, these symptoms will naturally heal on their own, since our body has an amazing way of bouncing back with plant-based nutrition, a positive mindset, meditation, supplementation, and simply slowing down.

Here are some silent signs of chronic inflammation inside your body:

- Joint and lower back pain
- Arthritis
- Active I.B.S, Colitis, Crohn's disease
- Constipation and toilet troubles
- Autoimmune disorders
- Belly fat & being overweight
- Acne
- Hormonal imbalances
- Eczema, Rosacea, Psoriasis
- High cholesterol
- High blood pressure
- Prominent visible wrinkles
- Bronchitis
- Heart disease
- Chronic pain
- Diabetes
- Easily ill with infections
- Mood disorders, anxiety, irritability
- Gallstones
- Gout

One of the times when I tested my ESR levels through a blood test (i.e. erythrocyte sedimentation rate, which is measurement of the level of inflammation in your body) was 45, which is very high (normal is between 1–15). When I was experiencing a Crohn's disease flare-up, my ESR was regularly in the high range.

After I had gotten sick and tired of being sick and tired, exhausted of being prescribed strong pills and potions, and being tube-fed and hospitalized all the time, my parents sought help from a well-known naturopathic doctor. This was life-changing to say the least — within a few months, my ESR was around 9, no joke! Today it rests between 7–9, and I get checked every few months to monitor my Crohn's disease.

My recovery came down to a few key changes: consuming natural nutrition from food, ditching wheat, gluten, dairy, and refined foods, adding a long list of life-supporting supplements, resting, and staying positive. To this day, lack of sleep, stress, and a diet dominated by inflammation-causing foods has huge impact on my health — if I give in to bad habits, I become unwell, sick, and very tired.

When your diet is based around meat, wheat, gluten, butter, cheese, milk, ice cream, refined sugar, alcohol, simple carbs(such as white bread), refined snacks, processed foods, and too much conventional meat, it can trigger the onset of inflammation; however, an abundance of plants can actually reduce your symptoms. When you start to heal your body holistically through natural nutrition, supplementation, and a positive mindset, it's amazing what the results are — I am living proof of this! Stress, lack of sleep, and poor eating habits put me right back in the hospital, and I feel weak and unwell again.

I am not saying I don't indulge every once in a while; however, the point is that if you are experiencing any of the symptoms listed above, commit to these nourishing foods. I assure that you can turbo-boost your health naturally by following the beauty food feasting list, and chances are, you won't have to resort to pills, and potions, that usually come with many side effects.

Beauty food feasting does not cure or treat; however, natural ingredients, especially plants, are highly healing, alkalizing, and nutrient-rich, and by consuming an abundance of plant-based foods (i.e. inflammation-fighting foods), you are likely to feel better physically, emotionally, and mentally.

By eating natural foods, you'll have a better chance to fight, address, and heal inflammation. Prevention is key to conquering chronic disease.

I am not against pharmaceuticals for a short-term solution, but natural remedies should be a part of your lifestyle first and foremost, so that hopefully, you won't have to resort to medication.

I haven't taken medication since my early 20s because I turn to natural remedies instead. When you eat natural forms of medicine in the form of food, you fill your body with vitamins, minerals, and antioxidants that help combat accelerated aging, oxidation in your cells from free radicals, and lifestyle-related illnesses. Combine this nourishment with meditation, mindfulness, a positive attitude, sunshine, fresh air, lots of water, supplementation, and you're golden.

I will forever be so grateful for my mother, who was hugely resourceful when it came to researching alternative therapies to help treat my Crohn's disease naturally. Google didn't exist yet, so there was no easy solution, yet she went out of her way to help me and wouldn't settle for what the doctors were doing, such as prescribing me pills that came with horrible side effects, including an immunosuppressant that could cause cancer and made me feel like I had the very bad flu — the doctors also suggested that I should have surgery to remove my bowels.

I am happy that I also have inherited my mother's trait of being a stubborn fighter who figures out other methods to become healthy and help others improve their health as well, especially when they are not feeling their best and are looking for other natural alternatives that may support them better than a typical short-term solution of pills and a poor diet.

Ashfab Living Tip: Do daily body scans when you wake up and before you go to sleep to check in with yourself. Are you in pain? Are you feeling low on energy? Are you suffering from tummy troubles? Are you bloated or breaking out with skin rashes, redness, or pimples? Are you feeling moody? These are imbalances in your body — pay attention to them before they get worse and lead to something more serious.

One of the reasons I was inspired to write this book is that I grew up with an illness, and I saw how nutrition and lifestyle played a key role in my recovery. I also witnessed close family members have strokes, suffer from painful arthritis, and be diagnosed with cancer — and they all had one thing in common: their diets were dominated by meat, wheat, milk, cheese, butter, and refined sugar, all of which were eaten because of tradition, convenience, and taste.

It was frustrating to see when the doctors didn't particularly give any valuable nutrition and lifestyle support, so since none of my family members made changes to their diets, they sadly did not heal or get better. Prescription drugs are for short-term solutions — I understand their usefulness; however, they usually treat the symptoms rather than getting to the root of the problem & treating the original cause of it. This is why I truly believe that people are better off reaching for natural foods to combat illness, while giving their body a range of nutrients to help their cellular health thrive. Again I am not saying diet and lifestyle can cure or treat chronic diseases however with a shift in healthy foods and habits, it can only bring benefits and hopefully help prevent future lifestyle related illnesses.

When members of my family were hospitalized from having a stroke, they were served white bread, butter, and things like cold-cut meats and cakes. I mean, really? They just had a stroke! Clearly their cholesterol or blood pressure was high, which is usually caused by too much saturated fat and trans-fats (meat, cheese, milk, and eggs are all high in saturated fat), and a heavy gluten-rich diet (which is highly inflammatory). If you consume plenty of plants and make other foods your sides or condiments, you can cut your risk of heart disease and certain cancers by a significant amount.

Even when I've been admitted to the hospital, I am served white bread, milk, concentrated juice, cheese, wheat, gluten, and sugary desserts — none of which are gut-friendly or contain enough fiber. It's no wonder that 300,000 people in the United States and over 200,000 in the UK suffer from bowel-related illnesses, as people are not really aware that nutrition and irritants play a role in health recovery.

On top of getting your ESR checked with a blood test, another great way to monitor your health at home is by measuring your pH levels on a regular basis. At 7.0, your body is healthy and alkalized, but if your reading is lower 6.0, you are very acidic, which is where disease and inflammation thrive. This might contribute to belly fat, headaches, fatigue, acne, skin rashes, hormonal imbalance, mood swings, high blood pressure, prominent wrinkles, and high cholesterol. Repeat the tests weekly to measure the improvements of the nutrition and lifestyle changes.

Beauty food feasting is highly alkalizing, so by consuming loads of leafy greens, fruit, berries, healthy fats, whole-grains, and other vegetables, you will see your pH level become healthier. The most acidic foods are mostly processed foods or animal products: meat, cheese, milk, eggs, coffee, alcohol, anything with gluten, cake, candy, cookies, crackers, and pretzels.

A food allergy test is also a mandatory step because if you are consuming foods that you are intolerant too, it can wreak havoc on your immune & reproductive systems, and it can disrupt your thyroid, mental health, and energy levels.

For example, I am sensitive to gluten and cow's milk. If I have them occasionally, I feel fine; however, if I consume these on a regular basis, I feel bloated, and blah, I may break out, in spots, don't sleep well, have brain fog, and feel moody and anxious — there's nothing beautiful about that at all.

As you continue on this wellness journey, pay attention to physical, mental and emotional symptoms. Do not ignore your body.

<u>Ashfab Health Tip: Use this testing checklist to monitor your inside health and to get to the root of any health, well-being, and beauty concerns holistically</u>

- **pH Balance:** measure your pH levels regularly. Shoot for a healthy range of 6.75–7.0. Anything under this range is highly acidic and is a recipe for disease and inflammation
- **ESR:** Get your ESR levels checked to see if you are experiencing inflammation. The healthy range is 1–10, and anything above 15 is a sign of internal inflammation.
- **Vega:** Schedule a Vega test to look for subtle abnormalities and imbalances. Usually treated with homeopathic remedies to heal naturally.

- **Food Allergy:** It is important to find out if there are any foods your body is intolerant to. This will play an important role in your waistline, energy levels, mental health, and skin condition. Eventually, you can consume these foods on occasion (unless you have Celiac disease, in which case gluten is completely off limits).
- **Blood Pressure & Cholesterol:** Check your blood pressure and cholesterol levels at least a few times a year, as these measurements are very important indicators of your health and longevity.
- **Bio-Resonance testing:** Bio-resonance testing is a non-invasive therapy that involves placing electrodes on your skin for diagnosis and treatment. The electrodes are connected to a "Bicom" machine that checks the energy wavelengths coming from your body, and then counteracts bad frequencies by restoring the optimum balance.

Yes, these scans and tests cost money; however, it's better to think of them as an investment in your well-being. Understand these imbalances before your symptoms get worse and chronic disease builds up in your body; prevention is key, and these types of tests are truly a window to your health.

Your body deserves to be treated with the best possible care, to be fed the best possible food, and to be cared for with the best love you can give. We only have one body and one life! We deserve to feel amazing and have tons of energy, glowing skin, and a strong body. We deserve to feel happy and balanced, and to have an unlimited capacity to exude vitality, radiance, and vibrant health. This is key to slowing down aging and increasing longevity.

If you think wellness is too expensive and not worth the investment, think of the hospital visits, medications, and missed work due to awful side effects and pain that you may experience in the future if you do not take care of your body. By making small changes to your health, you will reap the benefits and feel massive improvements from the inside out.

"Eating well is a form of self-respect and self-care."

Unknown

Natural nutrition is extremely inflammation-fighting, age-defying, and vitality-boosting. Again, I am not here to push a certain set of values regarding what you choose to eat. I am also not here to forbid foods or restrict your consumption. However, you will only experience amazing health, beauty, and well-being benefits when you focus on predominantly plant-based nutrition.

Try this plan for 10 days. Focus on feeling good, eating intuitively, and putting predominantly plant-based nutrition into your body. When you do, you will begin to naturally crowd out the foods that are not serving you or supporting your health, well-being, and beauty.

Don't overthink your meals or let yourself become rigid. The point is not to deprive or starve yourself; instead, be mindful and focus on feasting on beauty foods. It's not about what you can't eat — it's about the wonderful, nutritious foods you CAN eat. Shift your focus onto consuming nutrition and adding an abundance of delicious plants to your daily diet.

When you become a health conscious consumer, you will automatically choose the best and most fab foods to put in your body. The old you may want to scarf down that ham baguette with a soda pop and bar of chocolate, but the new you will ask yourself, "What is the most fab food to eat right now that will nourish my skin, cells, and spirit?

Remember, your inner health is a reflection of your outer health. Real foods will give you beautiful results. Think of it as turning to a more natural form of medicine that will improve your health and beauty.

I'm not saying this will be easy, but if you break it down into simple steps with simple reasons, you'll feel less overwhelmed. The goal is to learn to focus on what you **can** eat while reminding yourself that you are doing this for your health, well-being, and beauty.

Be gentle with yourself. During social gatherings, holidays, or special occasions, you may want to celebrate with your favorite treats. After you have followed a natural, mostly plant-based diet for a couple weeks, feel free to indulge a little. However, make sure to return to feeding your body a plethora of plants and natural nutrition most of the time.

The best part about adopting a new eating style is that you'll discover new, exciting flavors, experiment with seasonal ingredients, and learn to get creative in the kitchen. You'll inspire others around you to do so as well!

When you know that you are feeding your body the most fabulous foods, you will feel both inspired and empowered, especially when you see the fabulous results. It is entirely up to you how you choose to eat after you stick to the Ashfab nutrition plan. However, I can promise you this: your mind and body will thrive from implementing an abundance of plants, nuts, seeds, cold-pressed oils, fish and gluten-free grains, so why wouldn't you want to continue feeling amazing?

Ashfab Eating Tip: You will find a selection of recipes for each meal category. Simply follow the beauty food feasting guide, and experiment with the recipes provided. It's all about conscious, mindful eating that will nourish, energize, and turbo-boost your health.

As you learn to adopt healthier eating habits, it will become a natural instinct to feed your body healthy, fresh, natural nutrition. The more goodness you add to your diet, the easier it will be to naturally crowd out the not-so-good. If you don't have a lot of time, make the soups and salads in bigger batches so you can just grab-and-go, especially smoothies and juices are a great option since they can be made in minutes.

If you happen to have a social engagement in the next four weeks, try to modify and focus on the beauty food feasting list. It might be a good idea to write the main ideas in your notes so you'll always have it handy for reference.

Don't think of this as a diet; think of it as a lifestyle shift that you will continue to use every day and share with your loved ones. Feel a difference, see a difference, and be a whole new you.

Bye-bye bloat, aches, pains, spotty skin, and stress. Hello to the new you. Get in the routine of eating from the beauty feasting list. Focus on what you can eat, learn to get creative in the kitchen, use the seasonal shopping lists, and add herbs and spices to your dishes for extra flavour.

It's a good idea to start your day with a beauty booster shot to alkalize, cleanse, and detoxify your body. Begin every breakfast with a delicious plant-based smoothie that will give you a spectrum of nutrients. When you start the day healthy, chances are you will end it healthy. Enjoy a hearty salads or veggie sushi with greens for lunch, or perhaps a salmon bento box, a sumptuous soup, or with gluten-free oats topped with fruit or veggies.

For an afternoon snack, try a cold-pressed veggie-based vitality juice with handful of nuts, popcorn, or a plant-based protein bar.

For supper, look forward to a savoury feast of veggies with palm-sized protein or gluten-free wholegrain with veggies. Or maybe you'd prefer chunky soup, healthy tacos, gluten- and dairy-free casseroles, stew, or stir fry. Keep it fresh and simple, with natural nourishing ingredients — and boom! Call it a day.

Ashfab Eating Tip: Slow down during mealtimes, chew well, take small bites, eat from smaller plates, and savour the moment. Don't rush to eat! This is a sacred time to fuel your body and prepare for digestion.

Focus on beauty food feasting most of the time, leaving room for the occasional celebratory foods like red wine, dark chocolate, and other treats. When you are mindful of what your putting in your mouth, you naturally will gravitate toward the best options for your health.

You will also become more of a savvy shopper. Instead of choosing cows milk, you'll opt for plant-based milk. Instead of cereal, or sugary breakfast, you will start with a nutrient-rich smoothie. Suddenly, what felt daunting before will now be a positive habit that you have successfully implemented into your lifestyle. Add in the good stuff and crowd out the not-so-good stuff.

Once you adopt this style of eating and start feeling more energized, less bloated, and look like you're absolutely glowing, you will be more mindful about what you put on your plate.

Commit to this plan 100 percent for 10 days for maximum results, slowly build these new habits. Start with drinking a beauty tea after you wake up, and after a few days, add a plant-based breakfast smoothie to your routine. After that, start having plants for lunch & supper, and sip green juices religiously. Before you know it, you'll naturally adopt these healthy habits, and they'll become non-negotiable.

Ashfab Eating Tip: Allow yourself reward meals. This doesn't mean you can eat a whole deep dish pizza or apple pie all by yourself. Rather, save two or three meals if you like and eat them from a smaller plate. Eat slowly, take small bites, chew well, and savor the moment. Work toward finding healthier versions of your treat meals that are just as satisfying. Life is for living, so simply feed your body the most nourishing foods, and save room to celebrate with your favorite foods too.

Ashfab Health Tip for a Fab-Fix Recovery Plan: If you ever felt you overindulged over the weekend, which is okay, I would suggest spending the next day or two semi-fasting. Give your body a mini-break, aka holiday for your health!

The safest way to do this is to simply fill up on nourishing liquids all day along with 9–10 glasses of mineral water. Drink a health shot and sip a plant-based smoothie in the morning for meal times opt for sumptuous soups and 3-4 additional fresh veggies juices during the day. This will help you digest whatever is remaining in your body, relieve physical stress, and allow you to absorb and assimilate all the nutrients from the foods you consume. Instead of starving or punishing yourself, you are simply adding a whole lot of good stuff and getting rid of the bad to restore balance to your body.

I also do seasonal body boosts four times a year by applying this method over 3–4 days at the start of each season. This tradition helps me refresh and recharge my body to prepare it for the changing seasons.

Beauty Food Feasting Implements

Wellness Shot: Alkalizing, detoxifying, beautifying, cleansing, anti-inflammatory, anti-aging, anti-viral, and a potent anti-inflammatory, a wellness shot will set you up for an energizing, healthy day.

Smoothies & Juices: A daily ritual of drinking fresh juices and smoothies is one of the most effective and quickest ways to restore your health and get vital nutrients absorbed into your system quickly, which ultimately transforms your body and beauty from the inside out.

Soups: Soups are a great option nutritionally as they combine key nutrients, including vitamins and minerals that are nutrient-dense (high in nutritional value but low in calories). Get pure comfort from these delicious recipes that make great meals any time of the day.

Salads: Sumptuous salads bursting with vitamins, minerals, and antioxidants, are the perfect way to get a whole lot of nutrients in just one bowl

Sexy Suppers: Fabulous feasts that are bursting with fresh produce, fun flavors, and just the right amount of protein are easy and enjoyable to make in just minutes.

Sweet Treats: These sweet treats are a combination of healthy, delicious ingredients, and they're satisfying enough to fulfill your cravings.

Sexy Beauty Bowls: These bowls have a base of gluten-free whole-grains, like oats, quinoa, or teff made with nut milk and coconut oil or ghee, topped with berries, avocado, nuts, seeds, and maple syrup. They give you the perfect balance of healthy fats, plant protein, and complex carbohydrates. These are great for lunch, as they will satisfy you well until supper time.

Beauty Broth: These broths are highly nutritious, gut-healing, skin-loving, beautifying, inflammation-fighting, and rich in collagen.

BEAUTY FOOD FEASTING

Beauty food feasting begins with a fresh, energizing start to your day. Skip solid meals in the morning for a semi-fast: drink a wellness shot first thing, followed by a beauty-boosting smoothie. Come mid-day (noon +) have a nutrient rich lunch, then in the afternoon indulge in a large green juice with a small plant-based snack for an energy boost. In the evening, enjoy a satisfying supper packed with natural nutrition that is healthy, balanced, and varied.

Beauty Food Feasting: Daily Age-Defying Trio:

No matter what you have going on each day, try to implement a daily ritual of drinking the age defying trio, which will give you a spectrum of beautifying, health-boosting nutrients.

Wellness Shot

- Juice of 2 organic lemons

- Big pinch of turmeric
- Pinch of cayenne pepper * optional
- Good sprinkle of ground black pepper
- Drizzle of raw honey
- A little lukewarm mineral water

Glow-and-Go-Green Smoothie

- 2 types of leafy greens
- 2 berries
- 1 fruit *optional
- 1 scoop of plant protein powder
- Spoonful or 2 of super green powder
- Spoonful or 2 of a mixed superfoods powder as well as a spoon of mushroom base powder like Reishi

There are so many fabulous combos you can play around with, but the best thing is to start your day with a nutrient rich smoothie full of plant protein, fibre and healthy fats.

Vitality Juice

- kale
- spinach
- parsley
- cilantro
- lemon
- celery
- carrot
- beet

Either make your own, find an organic bar to prepare it for you, or pick up an organic veggie-based grab-and-go bottle with similar ingredients.

"A daily ritual of drinking a wellness shot, fresh smoothie, and nutritious juice is one of the quickest and most effective ways restore your health, well-being,

and beauty, transforming your body from the inside out naturally."

—Ashley Siedentopf

Beauty Food Feasting: Example Meal Guide

Morning

Elixir Beauty tea

- 1 juice of organic lemon
- 1 big pinch of turmeric
- 1 pinch of cayenne pepper
- Ground black pepper
- 1 drizzle of raw honey
- A little lukewarm mineral water

> * Recently for extra detoxifying properties I will make a small cup of detox tea. There are many brands on the market that have specific boxes of tea that are called DETOX with ingredients like dandelion, fennel and milk thistle in them. I let it steep for a few minutes, then add in the rest of the beauty blend.

Ashfab Beauty Shot Tip: Make a big batch of the elixir with five times the ingredients so you have it ready every morning during the week and simply add to the tea.

Breakfast

Create a fresh, home-made smoothie with the suggested ingredients. See recipes or scroll through @mrs.ashfab on Instagram for other smoothie ideas, or go visit the Ashfab Nutrition channel on YouTube.

Hydrate

Drink 8–10 glasses of mineral water. Add lemons for additional cleansing, detoxifying, and beauty benefits.

Mid-Morning

1 hot drink of your choice of matcha almond latte, oat flat white, herbal tea or whatever tickles your fancy.

Lunch

Enjoy a fresh, hearty soup or sumptuous salad, asian style soup and summer rolls, a gluten-free grain bowl with fresh toppings, a Japanese bento fish or plant based box, veggies dipped in fresh salsa and protein, eggs with avocado toast, or perhaps a gluten-free wrap with raw veg and sheep or vegan cheese.

Snack

Make or purchase an organic veggie juice (with no fruit except lemon) pair it with something like a plant-based protein ball, a handful of nuts, 1 cup of popcorn, or a gluten-free, sugar-free, dairy-free, whole grain muffin (make it at home or check organic bakeries and grocery stores). If you have a juicer, make two big batches on Sunday and in the middle of the week. Store them in air-tight jars in the fridge.

Even sipping on fresh raw juices just a few times a week can help get vital nutrients into your bloodstream, instantly giving you energy and alkalizing your system.

Supper

Cook sautéed veggies and serve plant-based or palm-sized lean organic protein. You could also make gluten-free wholegrains with veggies or choose from a selection of plant-based sushi. Other options include, chunky soup, omelettes, sumptuous salads, gluten-free grain pasta with your favorite nourishing sauce, wild-caught fish with generous amounts of sautéed greens or roasted root veg, veggie chilli, turkey chilli or tacos. I love mixing up modern Mediterranean-, Mexican-, and Asian-style suppers; these for me are the most satisfying and there are so many different options to cook with.

Dessert

Enjoy 1 cup of fruit, 2 squares of dark chocolate, dairy-free sorbet, or coconut yogurt with pomegranate, topped with hemp seeds and maple syrup. Sip on a cup of herbal calming tea, like Yogi Bedtime® tea. These are some things I love as a sweet treat, and sometimes i'll treat myself to a yummy frozen yogurt.

Ashfab Portion Control Tip: 1 serving = 1/2 cup, so aim for at least **7–9 servings** of fruits and vegetables per day through smoothies, snacks, superfood juices, soups, salads, and sides.

> **"Your state of mind affects your cellular health, so purify yourself from anger, guilt, resentment, worry, fear, jealousy and doubt."**
>
> **Unknown**

Beauty Food Feasting includes:

- Loads of leafy greens
- Root veggies, like parsnips, carrots, beetroot
- Colourful veggies
- Fruit, but fill up mostly on **berries** low in sugar and high in nutrients, antioxidants, and fibre
- Staple starches like sweet potato, beetroot, parsnips, and butternut squash
- Beans, legumes, pulses, and sprouts
- Superfoods like Maca, Acai, spirulina, Chlorella, wheat grass, moringa, reishi mushrooms, and ashwagandha
- Nuts and seeds
- Sea vegetables

- Healthy fats like coconut oil, avocado, ghee, and cold-pressed oils
- Hydrating liquids like mineral water, fresh veggie juices, and herbal teas
- Gluten-free whole-grains like brown rice, quinoa, gluten-free oats, gluten-free wholegrain bread, gluten-free wholegrain pasta, and gluten-free wholegrain wraps
- Plant protein like mushrooms, hemp seeds, tempeh, and occasional tofu
- Wild-caught organic salmon or white fish
- Raw honey, coconut honey, and pure maple syrup
- Bone broth (a few times a week), either homemade or organic store-bought

In Moderation

- Organic poultry & turkey
- Grass-fed and organic beef (only a palm-sized amount 1–2 x a week max)
- Small amounts of cheese made from sheep milk, like high-quality feta, halloumi, manchego, and pecorino
- Caffeine: 1-2 cup of premium coffee max per day with no cow's milk. Only consume after your health shot and smoothie.

Ashfab Eating Tip: If you choose to eat animal protein in moderation, look for organic, locally sourced meat.

Foods to Ditch, Reduce, or Eliminate for 10 Days

- Cow's milk: butter, milk, cheese, replace for plant based milks all together even after 10 days keep to a minimum or ditch altogether
- Highly processed refined foods: sugar cookies, chips or crisps, candy bars, crackers, cakes, fast food, white or brown bread, junk food. Do not keep this in the house. Make it extremely rare in your diet, as it will only hinder and deplete your health, beauty, and vitality

- Gluten: found in oats, barley, rye, wheat, soy sauce, stock, cereals, teriyaki, noodles, and pasta. Pay attention to labels, find gluten-free alternatives. Keep this to a minimum per the ashfab nutrition plan.
- **Pork**: after 10 days, consume seldomly
- **Soymilk**
- **Non-filtered tap water**
- **Cold-cut processed sandwich meats**
- **Margarine**

Ashfab Tip for Foods to Ditch: Photocopy this list, and either make sure it's visible or keep it with you. When you go shopping, focus your attention on natural nutrition, and ditch the food in bold altogether.

Alcohol

During the onset of your beauty food feasting journey, it is best to cut alcohol out completely, or to save it for rare, very special occasions.

Try to go alcohol-free for 10 days. Plan social engagements around healthy hangouts, and if it happens to be a busy time of year, choose high-quality red wine, premium tequila, premium gin and soda with limes, rose or white wine spritzers, or grain-free vodka and soda like Tito's or Cîroc. It's best to stay under 7 units during your first few weeks, but no alcohol at all is better, especially if you feel lots of toxins in your body.

If you choose to drink alcohol, stay hydrated. Drink a glass of mineral water between every drink. After 10 days, be mindful, and drink premium-quality alcohol in moderation. Hydrate twice as much as you normally do, and drink half as much as you did before. And remember: after every alcoholic beverage, drink one glass of mineral water.

Quick Color Guide

Foods in bold: reduce the foods in bold as much as possible, even after a few weeks. Find healthy alternatives for your favorite foods like nut milks, gluten-free wholegrain pastas, gluten-free wholegrain breads, vegan or sheep milk cheese. Simply focus on what you can eat and the beauty food feasting list.

Keeping your kitchen clear of any of the foods shown in bold makes it easier to stay on track. I am only human, and if I know there are Cheetos and Doritos in the house, you would see me inhaling both, at the same time LOL.

It's not that you can never have junk food again, but keeping it in the house is setting yourself up for disappointment. "Out of sight, out of mind" is a motto I live by, and it works.

Beauty food feasting nourishes your skin and heals and energizes your body. When you feed your body natural nutrition that is free from chemicals, gunk, and junk, and is ideally always locally sourced and organic, your body will thrive.

When you invest in your health and wellness, you feel better, are more productive, take fewer sick days, and have more energy for your loved ones, passions, and hobbies. Not to mention, you'll naturally balance out your body, so you can feel your best.

As you adopt a healthy attitude toward eating by drinking a health elixir upon waking, eating a nutrient-packed smoothie for breakfast, followed by a light lunch, a tasty glass of green juice, a small snack mid-afternoon, and a simple, savoury supper, your new habits will fall into place. When you start the day with something nourishing, you will most likely crave a healthy meal to end your day.

As I mentioned before, after you have completed the first 10 days in a row, it's then its safe to save 2–4 portion-controlled plates for a special time so that you can enjoy your favorite foods, but try to eat them over the weekend or break them up over the week for a couple of dinners. It's also a good idea to modify them as much as you can by making a healthier, beauty food feasting version of the meal (e.g. instead of going for a heavy carbonara, choose a small portion with a tomato base. Chew thoroughly, take small bites, eat slowly, and be mindful.

> **"90 percent natural, 10 percent naughty(ish) — this mindset not only empowers me to choose the most nutrient-dense foods to help nourish my cells, soul, skin and spirit; it also leaves no room for depriving myself from some of my favorite things."**

Back in my heyday (okay, I'm not THAT old — let's just say during my preteens), I remember considering the toppings on my cheeseburger (tomato and lettuce) as part of my five servings of fruits and veggies per day. In my mid-teens, the top-notch naturopath I was seeing told me that my diet needed an upgrade —although, my mum was actually quite good at making sure we had fruit as snacks and veggies at dinner. She even banned sugary cereals and soda pop! Those were a huge NO-NO in my household.

As you get older and become more "independent," you spend a lot of time going out with friends for lunch, dinner, or playdates. Although these activities revolve around food, it's not exactly "good" food most of the time.

The Standard American Diet, or S.A.D, is popular among many western-style cultures, which is unfortunate because fruit and veggie consumption is extremely low in these diets. So many people in today's world are overfed and under-nourished. It's no wonder that chronic illnesses and obesity are common among people who follow the S.A.D. — these illnesses stem from being deficient in nutrients and having a body full of toxins.

> **"Living a life of excess of consuming an imbalanced diet for extended periods of time can starve your body of the vitamins and other essential nutrients it needs to function."**
>
> **Unknown**

The Standard American Diet that many Western-style cultures follow looks something like this.

Breakfast: cereal, toast, or bagel, with concentrated juice and 2 cups of coffee with milk

Lunch: a sandwich, a granola bar, and a diet soda pop

Afternoon: chocolate bar, coffee, or another soda pop

Dinner: large portions of lasagna and cake

Whenever I go home to Canada and eat out, including my favourite hangout "Earls", *I go wild for their hot wings… nothing really compares lol*, however I am always surprised at how huge the portions are for a main dish in most of the restaurants. One portion back home would feed 2-3 people here in Europe. Anyhow my point here is to focus on eating the colours of the rainbow and from smaller plates, five servings of colourful fruits and veggies per day is usually the standard food guideline, but honestly, your body only really ends up absorbing not even half of what you eat, so I suggest eating between 7-9 servings a day. Now this number may seem a little ludicrous. You might be thinking, "Like, really, Ash? How do I have time to eat that many servings of fruits and vegetables in a day?" But before you go off on a rant, thinking, "oh, this can't be possible," know that it really is, and it becomes quite easy as you develop the habit of adding fruits and vegetables into all of your meals.

By doing so you are not only getting an abundance of fruit and veggies in your diet, but a plethora of vitamins, minerals, and antioxidants too, which boost your immune system, give you energy, aid digestion, and improve your mood, memory, and sleep quality. It will also help you naturally shed unwanted weight, especially around the tummy area, and it will give you glowing youthful skin, lustrous hair, and strong nails.

Eating the rainbow has amazing healing powers to help prevent and slow down accelerated aging and chronic illness. Many common illnesses today are food-related diseases. The people whose diets are dominated by plant-based nutrition have been shown to live longer, feel better, and look younger. Maybe now you are thinking, "Okay, so how do I do this?"

My Daily Beauty Feasting Routine

Here is an example of my daily beauty food feasting routine and how I get a whole lot of colour in my diet every single day.

> **"We cannot stop aging, but with predominantly plant-based nutrition, we can definitely slow the process down."**
>
> **—Ashley Siedentopf**

Morning

Elixir beauty tea: with juice of 2 lemons, turmeric, ginger, ground pepper, maple syrup or raw honey.

(2 serving)

Breakfast — 3-4 servings

Plant-based breakfast smoothie: 2-3 leafy greens, 1-2 berries, 1 fruit * optional, 1 scoop of vegan protein powder, ½ cup of coconut water or nut milk, scoop of mixed green powder, superfood blend and mushroom mix.

Lunch — 1-2 servings

Big salad, or fresh chunky veggie-based soup or veggies/ plant protein, topped over gluten-free grain, or veggies with a side of palm-sized protein, or Japanese bento box.

Snack/ large juice — 3-4 servings

500 ML of fresh green juice (kale, spinach, parsley, carrot, cucumber, celery, lemon) or veggie based and with a plant-based snack.

Hydration

8-9 glasses of mineral water

Supper — 2–3 servings

Sautéed veggies or raw veg with protein or gluten-free grain, chunky soup, or gluten-free pasta with fresh toppings, a casserole, stir fry or sumptuous salad.

As you can see, at the lower end of the spectrum, I could consume around 7–8 servings of fruits and vegetables a day, and at the higher, around 12. Remember: fruit and vegetables, especially leafy greens, are nutrient-dense so they contain a wealth of nutritional value with very few calories. This is why it's so important to make your diet predominantly plant-based, lots of nutrient rich ingredients for mega health and beauty benefits.

Tip: Drink a large glass of fresh, organic, green juice daily that was either cold-pressed, homemade, or store-bought, giving your body a plethora of vitamins, minerals, and antioxidants that are easier to digest, so you'll assimilate and absorb vital nutrients into your system quickly and turbo-boost your intake of at least 4–5 servings in a few gulps.

Tip: Add a premium green powder, a mushroom powder, and a mix of superfoods powder to your morning smoothies for maximum nutrition for alkalizing, detoxifying, and beautifying benefits.

For your body to fully thrive, you need to nourish it — not just occasionally, but on a daily basis with large amounts of vitamins, minerals, antioxidants, and phytonutrients from fresh, raw fruits and vegetables (ideally organic and locally sourced produce). By making plants a big part of your lifestyle, you naturally have more energy, better focus, and fewer sick days. You will also combat oxidation, which causes accelerated aging and lifestyle related illnesses.

I know it seems difficult to get a large supply of fruits and veggies in your daily diet; however, it is quite simple to implement smoothies, salads, soups, sides, and large quantities of fresh juice into your regime. When you flood your body with vitamins, nutrients, and live enzymes from raw fruit and veggies, you feel so good, it's hard to go back to your old habits. The side effects include glowing skin, better mood and memory, a slim waistline, strengthened immune system, and better digestion, just to name a few. Trust me on this!

I am a firm believer that it's what you do most of the time that matters in terms of eating, so focus on natural, simple, light, fresh, and colorful, rather than white, refined, meaty, rich, and heavy. What you do on a daily basis will affect your health, well-being, and beauty in a positive or negative way.

As I have mentioned before, the S.A.D. is dominated with foods like meat, dairy products, refined sugars, processed foods, refined grains, coffee, sugary drinks and alcohol. These types of foods are extremely acidic for your body, and not to mention, they are very toxic for your cells, organs, and overall health, which results in unwanted weight gain, disease, accelerated aging, and chronic illnesses.

When you fill your body with plenty of raw fruits and vegetables, it creates an alkaline environment. As I mentioned earlier, you should begin to monitor your PH levels. Anything less than 6.75 is extremely acidic, which means there is inflammation within the body. Strive for 7.0 for vibrant health, glowing skin, and loads of energy.

Loading up on plants helps cleanse and detoxify an acidic environment of years of damage. It truly is amazing how your body can heal and bounce back from natural nutrition. By having an abundance of fruits and vegetables, you will give your body the complete nourishment it needs to thrive.

As most of you know, deep, restful sleep is crucial for optimal health — this is something I discuss more in the next section. When you are snoozing away, you are actually in a natural state of detoxification, so what you put in your body first thing in the morning has a huge impact on your health, well-being, and beauty for the rest of the day. This is why I suggest starting your day with the beauty-boosting tea, followed by a nutrient-packed glow-and-go smoothie. By starting your day with these rejuvenating beverages, you are actually giving your body a small break and gently detoxifying your system daily to help it properly absorb and assimilate vital nutrients so your body can efficiently heal, digest, purify, cleanse, and strengthen your system from the inside out.

Eventually, you won't think of that buttered bagel, or bowl of cereal in the mornings; it's about creating new, healthy habits to crowd out other ones, and it naturally will become part of your lifestyle.

So How Do You Add the Rainbow to Your Diet?

Achieve amazing health and beauty benefits by consuming smoothies, salads, soups, large sides, big bases, fresh juices, and snacks.

I have compiled a list of the **five food color categories.** You don't need to like all of the fruit and veggies on this list, but there are so many, and it's a good experiment! Recently I have been loving radishes, and bok choy is something I didn't even think twice about eating just a year ago. Try something new, get creative in the kitchen and fill your plate with beautiful plants!

Your health will thank you for it today, and in the future.

Red & Pink

These pretty plants are rich in phytochemicals lycopene and anthocyanins that improve heart health and help decrease risk of certain types of cancers. They also boost circulatory, skin, and heart health.

- pink grapefruit
- tomatoes
- watermelon
- raspberries
- pomegranates
- strawberries
- cherries
- cranberries
- blood oranges
- beets
- radishes
- red peppers
- red apples

Yellow & Orange

These fruits and vegetables are coloured by beta-carotene, also known as Vitamin A, which helps fight free radicals from smoke, toxins, chemicals, and pollution and is amazing for skin and immune health.

- apricots
- gooseberries

- cantaloupe
- carrots
- yellow figs
- grapefruit
- lemons
- mangoes
- nectarines
- oranges
- papayas
- peaches
- yellow pears
- pineapples
- tangerines
- yellow beets
- sweet corn
- sweet potato
- yellow peppers
- butternut squash

Green

As you can probably guess, green produce gets its colour from a natural plant pigment called chlorophyll which is why they are called the king of the veggie kingdom. These plants, especially leafy greens, help cleanse and purify the blood and they're great for your skin, heart, gut, and immune health. These are the foods that are responsible for rejuvenation of your skin and body.

- avocados
- green apples
- green grapes
- green olives
- kiwi fruit
- limes
- green pears
- artichokes

- arugula
- asparagus
- broccoli
- Brussels sprouts
- chinese cabbage
- green beans
- celery
- cucumbers
- kale
- spinach
- collards
- mustard greens
- leeks
- lettuce
- green onion
- fresh peas
- green beans
- watercress
- courgette

Blue & Purple

These plants are coloured by natural pigments called anthocyanins that act as powerful antioxidants and protect cells from damage. Consuming blue and purple plants prevent accelerated aging, oxidation, bad moods, and memory loss. Add these daily to your morning smoothies, as they are essential properties for anti-aging and skin health.

- purple grapes
- blackberries
- purple plums
- prunes
- blueberries
- black currants
- black olives
- mulberries

- pomegranates
- aubergine

White

White produce is coloured by pigments called anthoxanthins that help lower cholesterol and blood pressure, and may help reduce the risk of certain types of cancers and heart-related diseases. They also boost immune health and vision.

- garlic
- onions
- parsnips
- shallots
- turnips
- cauliflower
- ginger
- mushrooms
- banana
- dates
- peaches
- brown pears

Now that you understand the variety of benefits that correspond with each colour, head over to your supermarket today, and opt for organic, locally sourced, seasonal ingredients for more flavour and nutrients.

Eat the rainbow to reap the benefits to feel and look fab today

The Importance of Organ Health

Keep your colon, liver, kidney clean for optimal health and beauty benefits. If you want to live longer, look younger, and feel better, pay attention to your liver, kidneys, and colon — these three organs can either hinder or help your health.

Signs of Poor Liver Function

If you have been neglecting your liver, it will not function well. Toxins and free radicals will build up, which will manifest as blemishes on your skin. It will also alter your hormones and cause unwanted weight gain.

Symptoms of a poorly functioning liver include:

- rosacea
- acne
- skin rashes
- spots
- saggy, itchy skin
- very visible wrinkles around the eyes

Keep in mind, nutrition plays a huge role in making the liver function optimally. A healthy liver will have an effect on your skin, giving you a clear, glowing complexion.

Foods That Boost Liver Function

Include liver-loving foods in your diet such as:

- beetroot
- parsley
- basil
- lemons
- turmeric
- avocado
- grapefruit
- nuts
- seeds
- most fruits and vegetables
- plant protein
- green juice
- gluten-free grains

- dandelion root
- milk thistle
- nettle herbs
- These foods and herbs will help protect and stimulate your liver. Although I love wine as much as anyone else, I must advise you to sip alcohol in moderation, and keep your toxic intake of processed or packaged foods to a minimum — your skin and scales will thank you for it.

Signs of Poor Colon Health

Your colon, also known as your gut, plays a huge part in your overall health and wellness. Poor digestion has both inner and outer signs and symptoms:

- bloating
- toilet troubles
- headaches
- abdominal pain
- foggy brain
- heartburn
- acid reflux
- blotchy skin
- breakouts around your chin, cheeks and forehead
- wrinkles
- frequent illness

When you reduce your intake of refined sugar, dairy, and gluten, it will have a profound effect on how you feel and look, as these ingredients massively compromise your colon, leading to many inner and outer symptoms.

Foods & Supplements to Boost Colon Health

Add gut-friendly foods and supplements to your diet to boost friendly bacteria and help promote a clean colon and clear skin. Foods and supplements you should consider adding to your daily routine are:

- aloe vera juice
- probiotics
- L-glutamine
- digestive enzymes
- flax seeds
- chia seeds
- gluten-free oats
- green leafy vegetables
- legumes
- bone broth
- blueberries
- bananas
- miso soup
- seaweed
- sweet vegetables, like sweet potatoes, beets, and carrots

Signs of Poor Kidney Health

Your kidney's main function is removing waste products from your blood and regulating water fluid levels. Even though these little bean shaped organs do not seem like an important part of your health, correlated problems often seem subtle, leading many people to neglect them.

Poor kidney function can cause an array of inner and outer signs and symptoms:

- difficulty urinating
- nausea or vomiting
- pain in your lower back or legs
- fatigue and lethargy
- puffy eyes

- under-eye bags
- prominent wrinkles around your eyes
- swollen feet, face, or hands

Tips to Boost Kidney Health

Firstly, it is vital to constantly cleanse your kidneys — meaning, drink up! I'm talking at least 2 litres of purified, filtered water daily. Personally, I love adding sliced lemons or cucumbers and berries to my water for added nutrients and taste, making it easier to sip. This will automatically improve kidney function, so if you suffer from any of those symptoms, they will diminish with daily water intake.

Secondly, compromised kidneys correlate to an acidic environment, meaning way too much refined sugar, processed and packaged foods, red meat, alcohol, coffee, cakes, cookies, crisps — basically, too much of anything you don't find in the produce section. Check the internet for many sources of alkaline and acidic food charts.

If you want to spring out of bed, feel energised, banish bloat, clear up your skin, boost your immunity, live longer, feel better, and look younger, take care of your kidneys, colon, and liver — they will thank you for it.

Ashfab Health Tip: Get a food allergy test! This is so important. If you have intolerances, they may be making you feel unwell, causing you to be over or underweight. This is because you will not be able to absorb vital nutrients, not to mention, you'll experience disrupted sleep, mood disorders, and anxiety.

Shop as much as you can in the produce section. Check labels for hidden ingredients, like refined sugar, gluten, wheat, cow's milk, chemicals, and artificial flavors. And don't forget to eliminate the foods in bold for at least 10 days.

Putting a Stop to Bloating

The word "bloating" seems to be popping up more and more these days (literally). Bloating is that uncomfortable feeling of swelling and tightness around your abdomen area, almost like there is a balloon inside you that has blown up and feels like it's ready to pop. It is one of the most common complaints among society today. Most people go undiagnosed for years, relying on pain medications and pills that wreak havoc on your digestion.

Having lived with Crohn's disease for 24 years now, I am the queen of debloating. Since my life involves many social engagements, airplane rides, and fun parties, I make sure I am prepared for the occasion throughout my day-to-day life.

Bloat Prevention:

Get Off the Gluten to rebalance from within

Some say it's a trend to cut gluten from your diet, especially if there seems to be no sign of a sensitivity or allergy. I would say remove it for a few weeks to see if it makes a difference on your gut health, then slowly reintroduce to see how you feel afterwards.

Gluten is a mixture of two proteins present in wheat, barley, rye, and oats. It is responsible for the elastic texture of dough, which is very hard to digest and break down, leading to — you guessed it — bloat.

Eliminate gluten from your diet, and choose gluten-free grains like amaranth, buckwheat, rice (brown or wild), millet, quinoa, teff, and whole grain pastas (but stay away from the corn ones if you can). Look for gluten-free wholegrain breads, which shouldn't be too difficult to find since there are so many on the market these days — just make sure they are not loaded with sugar.

Once you have abstained from gluten consumption for a while, it is perfectly okay to enjoy occasional pizza or pasta, sourdough toast, or to eat a pastry when you're out for dinner or on holiday; however, if you can reduce gluten most of the time, avoid stocking it in the house, and save it for special occasions, you will feel so much better! I'm all about natural nutrition with a hint of naughty, which makes me have a relaxed attitude towards eating and have a healthy relationship with food.

There are so many ways to swap ingredients for gluten-free options by getting creative in the kitchen. If you tend to have gluten in most of your foods, like corn flakes, Rice Krispies, other refined cereals, soy sauce, teriyaki sauce, some types of ketchup, refined porridge, rye bread, white and whole wheat bread, bagels, pasta, crackers, cookies, pretzels, beer, and vodka, you will most likely have bad bacteria in your small intestine, creating the perfect recipe for digestive problems, like bloating, discomfort, constipation, and cramps. In more severe cases, you might experience more severe digestive disorders like IBS, Crohn's disease, and colitis, as well as other mood disorders, anxiety, behavioural problems, and disrupted sleep.

If you are Celiac, however, you should definitely avoid gluten at all costs; but for most of us, abstaining most of the time is just fine. Again, don't stock gluten in your cupboards and read labels.

Most diseases and disruptions begin in the gut, physically, mentally and emotionally. Your gut health is connected to neurotransmitters in your brain; this is why one of the first benefits to beauty food feasting is feeling really happy, energised, and joyous. By removing or reducing gluten from your diet, you also keep wrinkles, pimples, and rashes at bay. If you suffer from eczema, psoriasis, rosacea, or acne, or if you are showing deep, prominent wrinkles, this will do your skin wonders.

Great gut health usually leads to wonderful overall health too. Try eliminating gluten for just 10 days, and you will see a massive improvement in your skin, immune system, digestive health system, mood, and memory.

Again, follow the beauty food feasting suggestions 100 percent, and then afterward, continue to base your meals on beauty food feasting guidelines, saving foods containing gluten for special occasions if you wish. To be successful, you'll need to become a food detective, looking for hidden gluten ingredients on labels and never stocking gluten in the house. Remember, gluten is usually found in wheat, oats, barley, and rye.

Bloat Prevention: Swap Cow's Milk for Plant Milk

Cow's milk is probably the biggest culprit of bloating. Ever indulge in a big ice cream sundae while you're on a date with your partner or pals, when suddenly, just minutes after taking your first bite, your jeans feel so tight, it is uncomfortable to sit?

Although many people do not realise it, most humans cannot digest cow's milk because of lactose. Lactose leaves undigested sugars in your colon, and as these sugars ferment, they cause bloating and cramping. Swap almond, rice, oat or hemp milk, and look for dairy-free alternatives to cheese, yogurts, and ice creams. It will make a world of difference, especially when you're on dates or out with friends.

If you're thinking, "Where the heck am I going to get my calcium from?" think again — you can get all the calcium you need by eating loads of leafy greens, consuming nut milks, and snacking on nuts and seeds. Cow's milk is not so great for our bodies and beauty — after all, it's for baby cows! — and consuming too much will only hinder your health. Trust me, when you remove it completely, you will notice the difference instantly. If you suffer from digestive problems like toilet troubles, bloating, cramping, pain, congestion, asthma, or skin issues like acne and eczema, removing cow's milk from your diet will have a profound effect.

Try the different types of plant milk to see which one you like. I recommend hemp milk, almond milk, rice milk, oat milk or coconut milk, all of which are very tasty and serve as a healthy replacement for dairy, with the added health and beauty benefits of the nut or plant. I love cheese, so I would never eliminate it completely. When I do crave cheese, I opt for cheese made from sheep's milk which is rich in protein and easy to digest. My favorite sheep's milk cheeses are manchego, pecorino, feta, and halloumi. Small amounts of dark chocolate (80 percent plus) is also permitted and has many health and beauty benefits.

Bloat Prevention: Reduce Refined Sugar for natural occurring ones like maple syrup, and raw honey.

There are many reasons for you to reduce your refined sugar consumption. Sugar consumption can have a disruptive effect on your blood sugar balance. It can contribute to cravings, excess weight gain, sluggishness, spotty skin, moodiness, and constant hunger.

However, one of the main reasons you should reduce your sugar consumption is because it can aid the onset of candida overgrowth and other harmful micro- organisms. Candida overgrowth is increasingly associated with many diseases, including small intestinal bacterial overgrowth (S.I.B.O.).

If you want to learn more about the dangers of refined sugar, I highly recommend reading "Sugar Blues" by William F Duffy, the classic, best-selling exposé on the bad effects of sugar reveals how this commonly ingested ingredient in countless foods is highly addictive and causes a host of medical problems, from depression to coronary thrombosis.

Bloat Prevention: Get that Digestive System Moving

Often people think that going to the restroom a few times a week is normal, but it doesn't have to be. I've been on both sides of the spectrum, from frequent trips to less frequent, so I can relate really well to the less frequent. When I lived in Italy for a year and had a diet full of pizza, pasta, and gelato, let me tell you, I felt like one big turkey gobbling and hobbling around Milan.

Constipation is not only a silent killer, but its biggest symptom is constant bloating. If this sounds like you, try out a four-day juice cleanse to help your bowels start moving and working again. Be sure to include loads of fresh produce that is rich in fiber. Add high-fiber plant-based soups, salads, snacks, smoothies, and super juices to your diet.

For extra help getting things moving, drink a big cup of pure aloe vera juice, take magnesium oxygen daily, sip liquids like herbal teas and fresh juices, and load up on filtered water. Drink at least half your weight in ounces, and make sure you are doing daily trips to the toilet. Bye-bye bloat, hello flat tummy!

Bloat Prevention: Eliminating Bad Bacteria With Probiotics

Taking premium probiotics 50 Billion +, has profound effects on your gut health. It helps balance out your digestion to boost the good bacteria in your gut. If you have an overgrowth of bad bacteria, your gut health will be out of whack, which will inevitably cause you to bloat.

Fixing your gut bacteria also boosts your mood and mental health. It will help you shift weight easier and banish the bloated look — combined with beauty food feasting, you'll get a flat tummy in no time. Probiotics will also help give you a clear, flawless complexion. This supplement will also boost your immune system and make digestive disorders like Crohn's disease, colitis, and I.B.S, more manageable.

Take probiotics daily to experience a significant effect on your digestion. You'll banish your bloat and feel lighter, brighter and less bloated.

Bloat Prevention: Pop the Bubble Belly With Peppermint

Peppermint tea is one of my go-to herbal teas that is not only refreshing, tasty and invigorating, but extremely effective for de-puffing and banishing bloat. It is a great drink any time of the day, but if you are feeling more bloated than usual, make a potent pot of peppermint tea, around 3–4 bags, and sip within an hour. Do this several times a day, and watch the swelling go down. Another option is to rub pure organic peppermint oil all over your belly, followed by a hot cloth compress on top.

Bloat Prevention: Book a Colonic Treatment

If you have suffered from bloating, discomfort, and general tummy troubles for a long period of time, I would suggest booking in a colonic treatment with a trained therapist to give your colon a good cleaning, remove all that bad bacteria, and boost your overall gut health. When you have good gut health, you are able to assimilate and absorb nutrients much better, which is beneficial for your overall health, well-being, and beauty. As I have crohns disease I have to stay away from colonics, however my fellow wellness advocates rave about them, and cannot get them however if i could, I would totally be on board. So for those with sensitive tummy like me, try oral style cleaning like gulping a big glass of aloe vera juice over a few days, with magnesium oxygen citrate 500 mg before bed….. instant flush.

Bloat Prevention: Chew Your Food Thoroughly & Slowly

Chewing your food slowly is a very important factor in helping you feel less bloated and uncomfortable. It is really important to chew your food thoroughly and simply slowing down when you are eating your meals.

Take your time to enjoy the taste and flavours, and be mindful of that moment. Your body begins the digestion process while you chew, as your saliva breaks down your food and absorbs nutrients. Mindful eating is both meditative and nourishing.

Next time you begin your meal, start by being grateful for the food on your plate, and simply take your time to enjoy the meal to the very last bite. Not only will it do your body and bloat good, you'll also feel full more quickly. One thing I have noticed over years of studying nutrition and seeing clients who often struggle with keeping the weight off is they eat about twice as much as they need to, and they eat about twice as fast. Slow down, chew well, and eat off of smaller plates if it helps. You will notice a big difference in your bloat since you are not putting so much stress on your digestive system.

Bloat Prevention: Extra Good Stuff

To really beat that bloat and maximize a healthy diet full of plants, take 400 -500 mg of magnesium citrate or oxygen, with night spray, drink a large glass of pure aloe vera juice a day, and add healthy fats from coconut oil, avocado, or cold-pressed oils to your salad to help move the fiber swiftly in your bowel.

Bloat Prevention: Nasty Lil' Things

If you're constantly bloated, always tired, wiped out with constant infections, wake up often in the night, suffer from frequent constipation, suffer from skin redness, rashes, rosacea, can't seem to shift your muffin top, it is worth getting tested for parasites. It may sound a little icky, but hey, if you have travelled internationally, eaten something slightly uncooked meat, or uncleaned fruits and vegetables, it just takes one time for the little creature to make its way to into your system, leaving you not feeling so great!

Try to find a well-known practitioner in your area who does Vega testing, as discussed in the previous section to detect worms, parasites, and other unknown imbalances, as well as a comprehensive stool sample test.

The reason I wanted to touch on the topic of bloating even though beauty food feasting really helps alleviate symptoms, bloating is something that so many people suffer from it, so they just keep resorting to pills and potions to de-bloat, but they never actually heal and repair the problem. That's why I say that you should really dedicate at least 10 days to eliminating the bold food list, and while you're at it, thoroughly chew your food, slow down at mealtimes, and eat off of smaller plates.

> **"I am no saint, and I am as indulgent as I am disciplined. I enjoy smoothies, sumptuous salads, and green juices, as much as I enjoy devouring a decadent dessert, sipping on some pinot noir, or occasionally, savoring fresh sourdough pizza. It's all about balance because balance compliments a healthy lifestyle. If I feel I have overindulged, I will make sure to double up on healthy goodness the following days, and I'll add some additional sweat sessions while doing a fab semi-fasting fix."**
>
> **- Ashley Siedentopf**

I try to adopt healthy habits like intuitive eating, a positive mindset, meditation, and daily movement, while also following a diet dominated by natural nutrition. This type of lifestyle works wonders for me, as it takes away any feelings of guilt and deprivation for my favourite things in life. Focus on all the good stuff that makes you feel great to save room for treats that you love.

Simply focus on beauty food feasting, and after 10 days of total commitment, continue to make this as part of your lifestyle, occasionally treating yourself to treats if you fancy them. You will look and feel so good that beauty food feasting will become a normal part of your daily routine. Add in the good stuff to crowd out the bad stuff, and learn to get confident and creative in the kitchen. Focus on planning your meals around plants, eat off smaller plates, chew slowly, and save room for treats you really enjoy occasionally. Life is for living, after all, and yes, you should have that slice of cake if you want it.

Moderation in Moderation

Soon, it will become a habit naturally to start your morning with a wake-up wellness shot, sip on nutrient-packed smoothie to set your day for success. You'll enjoy a healthy lunch packed with predominantly plant-based ingredients, like a sumptuous salad, chunky soup, sushi, or gluten-free oat bowl, followed by afternoon energy-boosting veggie juice as a small snack, and by supper time, you'll devour some veggies with a side of plant protein or gluten-free grains, or maybe you'll feast on wild-caught fish or generous seasonal sautéed greens with a side of grass-fed beef. When in doubt, just keep it simple, fresh, and natural — don't over complicate it.

After living in places like France, Italy, and Greece, I noticed that they all have something in common: they consume fresh natural foods and still enjoy the finer things in life like sipping wine, grazing cheese, nibbling on dark chocolate or something sweet, and they seem to live long healthy lives.

I am human too, and sometimes, I want a good-quality cheeseburger, piping hot sourdough pizza, or a skinny margarita (or 2 or 3), but my diet is dominated by natural nutrition. I focus on an abundance of plants, eating smaller portions, and eating slowly. By doing this, I have healed my struggle with Crohn's disease naturally, I feel 10 years younger, and I've maintained a healthy weight consistently for years now — not by restricting myself, but by choosing the best foods to boost, balance, and beautify my body from the inside out, knowing when to use supplements to help my cells thrive. I rock a positive attitude, have an optimistic mindset, and I move my body daily, always focusing on feeling good.

When you really commit to this, you are doing something for you and your body, and the first thing you'll notice is the feeling you get from doing this. When I overeat things that are processed, not-so plant-based, rich in gluten, full of dairy or refined sugar, I feel extremely bloated, and instantly lose my glow. The foods I consume have a powerful effect on both my inner and outer beauty. You are what you eat, digest, and absorb — most of the time. No, you will not feel bad and look bloated if you indulge in small treats on occasion. It's what you are doing most of the time that will have the biggest impact on your health, wellbeing and beauty. If you consume 21 meals per week, you can still have 2–3 treat meals spread out over a 7-day period because you are still consuming 18 nutrient-packed ones — that's a whole lotta good sh** you're putting in your body! Hoorah for that!

Don't follow diets that are about calorie counting, deprivation or strict rules. A healthy balance is realistic and way more sustainable. Focus on the beauty feasting guide I have given you, use the shopping lists every season, and you will naturally grow into the fabulous person you deserve to be, from the inside out.

If you feel you have slipped back to old habits again, simply pick this book up again for an inner-outer beauty boost to remind yourself of the Fab formula tips.

> **"Making healthy choices makes me feel good. When I don't move my body enough, become lazy, and eat too much junk food, I feel bloated, lethargic, and just blah! I prefer feeling light, healthy and happy."**
>
> **—Ashley Siedentopf**

Eat off of smaller plates, take small bites, savour your senses in the moment, and chew well. When you eat fast, you don't feel full, which will cause you to eat more than your body actually needs. Take your time when you eat your meals — enjoying beautiful food is a sacred moment. After you have completed the plan, make a pact, and set an intention to choose meals that are dominated by an abundance of plants for fabulous health, well-being, and beauty benefits. "Our health is our wealth," so invest in yourself now.

The most important thing is knowing that putting the best, nourishing, natural nutrition in your body will make you feel and look your best. You will become more conscious and mindful, which will help you avoid binge-eating or reverting to poor eating habits. Remind yourself! This is for you! And you want to be here, feeling and looking your best, for as long as possible.

By having a diet dominated by natural nutrition, an abundance of plants, and healthy choices, you will feel empowered, and when your loved ones see the benefits, they'll be inspired to do the same.

Fill your plate with natural nutrition that makes you look and feel pretty, treat yourself to cravings in moderation after the first few weeks, and be proud of yourself for choosing vibrant health. Notice and feel the results you get when you feed your body with real, natural, plant-based nutrition.

Being a health and wellness advocate takes dedication, discipline, devotion, and knowing that you are only gaining inner and outer beauty benefits is motivation itself.

After you follow the meal plan for 10-days, congratulate yourself for the new path you have carved towards optimal health and wellness. Be conscious of your choices, switch to a beauty food mindset, focus on nourishing your body with natural nutrition, and you will feel empowered and inspired to put you, your health, and your body first.

The key to long-term success is simply using the Beauty Food Feasting Guide as a base. Make it a habit to drink the elixir wake-up wellness shot first thing, followed by a homemade plant-based green smoothie and a large glass of veggie-based cold-pressed juice in the afternoon. Adding additional fresh veggie juices is another way to dominate your diet with plant-based nutrition. By doing so, you are giving your body a plethora of important vitamins, minerals, and antioxidants that will help combat oxidation. Oxidation accelerates aging and lifestyle-related illnesses.

Consuming phytochemicals (plant-based nutrition) will help your body fight off the harmful effects of oxidation, keeping your cells and enzymes happy and healthy, your energy levels high, your waistline slim, and your skin glowing and radiant.

Make yourself a priority and set a daily intention to live your most fabulous life possible. That means eating and feeding your most fabulous self with nourishing foods that will naturally want to choose foods from the *Beauty Food Feasting Guide* and keep crap out of the house.

If you become obsessive with calorie counting and eating clean daily, you'll create an imbalance from within, Instead, simply make healthy choices, treat yourself sometimes, and find a happy balance for your well-being, beauty, and body.

"Once you have completed the 10-day challenge and implemented beauty food feasting into your life, allow cocktails, cronuts, or cupcakes to be special treats instead of your source for fuel."

—Ashley Siedentopf

To start this transformative lifestyle solution, do a major kitchen declutter — throw out gluten rich ingredients, cow's milk, and processed foods or refined foods. Afterward, fill your fridge with seasonal fruit, veggies, nuts, seeds, gluten-free grains, and mineral water, and stock your pantry with nuts, seeds, cold-pressed oils, wild fish, and superfoods. Use this fab food shopping list each season!

Eating healthy and staying healthy also means eating seasonal and local produce. By choosing in-season foods, you will benefit from maximum nutrition; at least three times more vital nutrients are found in local, seasonal crops. You also support local farmers, and the taste of the produce is much more delicious since the fruits and veggies have fully ripened and kept their flavour.

Organic, Seasonal Foods Are Better for Your Health

When fruits and vegetables are picked at their peak and grown locally and organically, they will have triple the nutrients that non-local, non-organic produce has — and four times the flavour! Eating organic, seasonal produce is also the best way to eliminate the harmful effects of pesticides on your health. Food grown without chemicals is the best way to feed your body.

Organic, Seasonal Eating Supports Local Farmers & Helps the Environment

More than likely, your food is grown locally, or at least regionally, when it's in-season, meaning there are less emissions required to send it your way. It also takes less energy and effort to grow foods in their ideal climate and growing conditions, which means your food consumption leaves a smaller ecological footprint.

Organic Seasonal Eating Means More Colourful, Fun, Fab Variety

It's easy to opt for the same weekly choices that you and your family are familiar with, like potatoes, corn, and carrots. However, when you use my fabified shopping lists, you will end up adding more colour, variety, and fun ingredients to your cart. This means you'll be getting a little more creative in the kitchen. You'll be eating new things, full of fab flavor, every season, and the fun food choices will make meals more interesting and healthier.

Make a few copies of the shopping lists below and have them handy when you go to the store.

Fabified Shopping List — Summer

Gluten-Free Whole-grains

- *Gluten-free* oats
- Quinoa
- Millet
- Spelt
- Brown rice
- Popcorn
- Teff
- Rice Cakes
- *Gluten-free* Wholegrain Bread, Pasta or Wraps

Fruit

- Apricots
- Asian Pear
- Barbados Cherries
- Black Currants
- Blackberries
- Blueberries
- Boysenberries
- Breadfruit

- Cantaloupe
- Casaba Melon
- Champagne Grapes
- Cherries
- Crenshaw Melon
- Durian
- Elderberries
- Figs
- Grapefruit
- Grapes
- Honeydew Melons
- Jackfruit
- Key Limes
- Limes
- Loganberries
- Longan
- Loquat
- Lychee
- Mulberries
- Nectarines
- Passion Fruit
- Peaches
- Persian Melon
- Plums
- Raspberries
- Sapodillas
- Sapote
- Strawberries
- Apples
- Watermelon

Vegetables

- Beets
- Bell Peppers
- Butter Lettuce

- Chayote Squash
- Chinese Long Beans
- Corn
- Crookneck Squash
- Cucumbers
- Eggplant
- Endive
- Garlic
- Green Beans
- Green Soybeans
- Jalapeño Pepper
- Lima Beans
- Manoa Lettuce
- Okra
- Peas
- Radishes
- Shallot
- Sugar Snap Peas
- Summer Squash
- Tomatillo
- Tomatoes
- Winged Beans
- Zucchini

Lean Protein

- Organic or locally sourced lamb
- Organic chicken
- Grass-fed beef
- Cod
- Crab
- Mackerel
- Salmon
- Dover Sole
- Sea bass
- Shrimp

- Halibut
- Scallops
- Prawns
- Sardines

Hydrating Liquids

- Natural Mineral Water
- Fruit-Infused Purified Water
- Herbal Teas
- Freshly Made Vegetable Juices.

Healthy Fats

- Coconut Oil
- Extra Virgin Olive Oil
- Avocado
- Sesame Oil
- Olives
- Basil Oil

Nuts & Seeds

- Almonds
- Cashews
- Hazelnuts
- Mixed Nuts
- Peanuts
- Peanut Butter
- Pecans
- Pistachios
- Pumpkin Seeds
- Sesame Seeds
- Sunflower Seeds
- Walnuts

Beans & Legumes

- Adzuki
- Black Beans
- Black-Eyed Peas
- Chickpeas
- Falafel
- Kidney Beans
- Lentils
- Lima Beans
- Navy Beans
- Pinto Beans
- Soybeans

Superfoods

- Acai
- Baobab
- Bee pollen
- Cacao Nibs
- Camu
- Cayenne Pepper
- Chia Seeds
- Chlorella
- Ghee
- Hemp Seeds
- Kefir
- Nutritional Yeast
- Maca
- Mangosteens
- Spirulina
- Turmeric

Fabified Shopping List — Autumn

Gluten-Free Whole Grains

- Gluten-free oats
- Quinoa
- Millet
- Spelt
- Brown Rice
- Popcorn
- Teff
- Gluten-free grain bread
- Gluten-free Wholegrain Pasta or Rice Pasta

Fruit

- Asian Pear
- Barbados Cherries
- Cactus Pear
- Cape Gooseberries
- Crab Apples
- Cranberries
- Feijoa
- Grapes
- Guava
- Huckleberries
- Key Limes
- Kumquats
- Muscadine Grapes
- Mushrooms
- Passion Fruit
- Pear
- Pineapple
- Pomegranate
- Quince
- Sharon Fruit

- Sugar Apple
- Vegetables
- Acorn Squash
- Belgian Endive
- Black Salsify
- Broccoli
- Brussels Sprouts
- Butter Lettuce
- Buttercup Squash
- Cauliflower
- Chayote Squash
- Chinese Long Beans
- Delicata Squash
- Daikon Radish
- Endive
- Garlic
- Ginger
- Jalapeño Peppers
- Jerusalem Artichoke
- Kohlrabi
- Pumpkin,
- Radicchio
- Sweet Dumpling Squash
- Sweet Potatoes
- Swiss Chard
- Turnips
- Winter Squash

Lean Protein

- Organic or locally sourced lamb
- Organic Chicken
- Cod
- Crab
- Mackerel
- Salmon

- Dover Sole
- Sea bass
- Shrimp
- Halibut Scallops
- Prawns
- Sardines

Healthy Fats

- Coconut Oil
- Extra Virgin Olive Oil
- Avocado
- Sesame Oil
- Olives
- Basil Oil

Nuts & Seeds

- Almonds
- Cashews
- Hazelnuts
- Mixed Nuts
- Peanuts
- Peanut Butter
- Pecans
- Pistachios
- Pumpkin Seeds
- Sesame Seeds
- Sunflower Seeds
- Walnut

Beans and Legumes

- Adzuki
- Black Beans
- Black-Eyed Peas
- Chickpeas

- Falafel
- Kidney Beans
- Lentils
- Lima Beans
- Navy Beans
- Pinto Bean
- Soybeans

Superfoods

- Acai
- Ashwagandha
- Baobab
- Bee Pollen
- Cacao Nibs
- Camu
- Cayenne Pepper
- Chia Seeds
- Chlorella
- Ghee
- Hemp Seeds
- Kefir
- Nutritional Yeast
- Maca
- Mangosteens
- Reishi
- Spirulina
- Turmeric
- Wheat Grass

Fabified Shopping List — Winter

Gluten-Free Whole Grains

- Gluten-free oats
- Quinoa

- Millet
- Spelt
- Brown Rice
- Popcorn
- Teff
- Gluten-Free Grain Bread

Fruits

- Clementine's
- Dates
- Grapefruit
- Kiwifruit
- Mandarins
- Oranges
- Passion Fruit
- Pear
- Red Currants
- Tangerines

Vegetables

- Belgian Endive
- Brussels Sprouts
- Butternut Squash
- Collard Greens
- Squash
- Kale
- Leeks
- Sweet Dumpling Squash
- Sweet Potatoes
- Turnips
- Winter Squash

Healthy Fats

- Coconut Oil
- Extra Virgin Olive Oil
- Avocado
- Sesame Oil
- Olives
- Basil Oil

Lean proteins

- Organic or Locally Sourced Lamb
- Organic Chicken
- Cod
- Crab
- Mackerel
- Salmon
- Dover Sole
- Sea bass
- Shrimp
- Halibut
- Scallops
- Prawns
- Sardines

Nuts & Seeds

- Almonds
- Cashews
- Hazelnuts
- Mixed Nuts
- Peanuts
- Peanut Butter
- Pecans
- Pistachios
- Pumpkin
- Seeds

- Sesame seeds
- Sunflower Seeds
- Walnuts

Beans and Legumes

- Adzuki
- Black Beans
- Black-Eyed Peas
- Chickpeas
- Falafel
- Kidney Beans
- Lentils
- Lima Beans
- Navy Beans
- Pinto Beans
- Soybeans

Superfoods

- Acai
- Ashwagandha
- Baobab
- Bee Pollen
- Cacao Nibs
- Camu
- Cayenne Pepper
- Chia Seeds
- Chlorella
- Ghee
- Seeds
- Kefir
- Nutritional Yeast
- Maca
- Mangosteens
- Reishi

- Spirulina
- Turmeric

Fabified Shopping list — Spring

Gluten-Free Grains

- Gluten-free oats
- Quinoa
- Millet
- Spelt
- Brown Rice
- Popcorn
- Teff
- Gluten-free grain Bread
- Whole grain pasta

Healthy Fats

- Coconut Oil
- Extra Virgin Olive Oil
- Avocado
- Sesame Oil
- Olives
- Basil Oil

Fruit

- Apricots
- Barbados Cherries
- Bitter Melon
- Honeydew
- Jackfruit
- Limes
- Lychee
- Mango

- Oranges
- Pineapple
- Strawberries

Vegetables

- Artichokes
- Asparagus
- Broccoli
- Butter Lettuce
- Cactus
- Chayote Squash
- Chives
- Collard Greens
- Corn
- Fava Beans
- Fennel
- Green Beans
- Manoa Lettuce
- Mustard Greens
- Pea Pods
- Peas
- Purple Asparagus
- Radicchio
- Ramps
- Red Leaf Lettuce
- Rhubarb
- Snow Peas
- Spinach
- Spring Baby Lettuce
- Swiss chard
- Watercress

Nuts & Seeds

- Almonds

- Cashews
- Hazelnuts
- Mixed Nuts
- Peanuts
- Peanut Butter
- Pecans
- Pistachios
- Pumpkin Seeds
- Sesame Seeds
- Sunflower Seeds
- Walnuts

Beans and Legumes

- Adzuki
- Black Beans
- Black-Eyed Peas
- Chickpeas
- Falafel
- Kidney Beans
- Lentils
- Lima Beans
- Navy Beans
- Pinto Beans
- Soybeans

Superfoods

- Acai
- Ashwagandha
- Baobab
- Bee pollen
- Cacao Nibs
- Camu
- Cayenne Pepper
- Chia Seeds

- Chlorella
- Ghee
- Hemp Seeds
- Kefir
- Nutritional Yeast
- Maca
- Mangosteens
- Reishi
- Spirulina
- Turmeric

Herbs & Spices

- Turmeric
- Garlic
- Sea Salt
- Black Pepper
- Oregano
- Parsley
- Basil
- Chili Flakes
- Paprika
- Cinnamon
- Cardamom

Suggested Supplements & Product Essentials

Invest to maximize your health, well-being, and beauty.

- **Premium Probiotics (~50 Billion +)** this will boost the good bacteria in your gut, it also helps with clear skin, reducing tummy troubles, strengthening your immune system, and improving your mood
- **Magnesium Citrate (400 milligrams or Spray):** Use before bedtime to calm your nervous system.
- **Omega-3:** for skin, hair, immune, brain, and heart health

- **Vitamin C Spray or Supplement:** helps combat oxidation and fights free radicals
- **Digestive Enzymes:** eat with each meal to help absorb and assimilate nutrients properly
- **Vitamin D:** if you do not live in a sunny climate, you are likely to be deficient, so it's important to get Vitamin D from food and supplements, if you live in colder conditions take 40k IU a week during the colder months and 10-20k IU spring / summer
- **Vitamin B-100:** for mood and memory
- **Plant-Based Protein Powder:** add this powder to your morning smoothies to maximize nutritional benefits. Great products include Vega One® and Garden of Life RAW Organic Protein
- **Organic Whole-Foods-Based Multivitamin:** one product I love is Garden of Life Daily Women Multivitamin

- **Extra, Optional Investments for Your Liver & Colon**

- **Milk Thistle:** supports your liver. You might not need it all year long, but it is a good idea to take one or two bottles at each seasonal onset. This will help you cleanse extra built up fat and toxins.
- **Aloe Vera Juice:** sip a big glass of aloe vera juice every day, in the morning or before bed, for massive colon-cleansing effects and gut-healing benefits. Highly healing for gut and skin health.

- **Guide to Superfoods & Their Benefits**

Superfoods are highly nutritious, and all come with many different health-boosting and beautifying benefits add them to smoothies, soup or salads or take as supplements.

Acai: Contains high levels of antioxidants. Boosts energy, curbs cravings, contains cancer-fighting agents, and provides amazing antiaging and skin benefits

Ashwagandha: Reduces stress and anxiety, has calming effects, rejuvenates vitality from within, boosts fertility, and balances blood sugar levels

Baobab: Rich in Vitamin C. Boosts your immune system, delivers a slow energy release, improves skin health, and helps absorb iron

Bee Pollen: Rich in Vitamin B. Improves mood, memory, brain function, energy, and alertness

Cacao: Contains the highest levels of antioxidants on this planet and is the highest plant-based source of iron. Boosts your mood and uplifts your happiness from within

Camu: Rich in Vitamin C. Reduces inflammation and fights or prevents viruses and bacteria

Cayenne Pepper: Boosts digestion, soothes irritation, speeds up metabolism, and detoxifies the body

Chia Seeds: Rich in omega-3 fatty acids. Improves skin, brain function, and heart health. Contains lots of fiber to help you stay fuller for longer

Chlorella: Rich in iron. Boosts energy, curbs cravings, improves skin, and gives a clear, glowing complexion

Ghee: Rich in Vitamin A, E, & K. Improves digestion and helps you feel full. Has incredible healing properties and is great to add in oatmeal or to use in cooking

Hemp Seeds: Rich in omega-3 and -6. Lowers blood pressure and cholesterol. Great source of plant protein. Improves figure and boosts skin health

Nutritional Yeast: Rich in B vitamins and Zinc. Has a nutty, savory, cheesy flavor that gives more flavor to vegan dishes. Fights oxidation, boosts immune system, and lowers cholesterol

Maca: Boosts energy and fertility health. Increases stamina. Improves mood and reduces depression, anxiety, and adrenal stress

Mangosteen: Improves menstrual health & skin health. Aids tummy troubles and digestion problems

Reishi Mushroom: Promotes longevity, fights infection, prevents and combats cancer, boosts mood, and fends off depression

Spirulina: Contains high levels of iron and Vitamin B. Boosts energy, detoxifies the body, and promotes a glowing, clear complexion

Turmeric: Natural medicine that heals the body, reduces inflammation, prevents and fights viruses, detoxifies the body, and contains antioxidants

Meal Ideas

Food combinations that will make you feel great, and look great

Eating well comes down to proper planning, smart shopping, and meal prepping. Once you get the hang of it, you soon will be on your way to healthy eating that is easy-to-make and tasty. Opt for organic and locally sourced ingredients whenever possible.

Smoothies to Boost Your Health & Beautify Your Skin

The general idea is to use 1–2 types of berries and 1–2 leafy greens as your smoothie base, then add other fruits and superfoods that you love.

Cocoberry

- 1 large handful of blueberries
- 1 large handful of raspberries
- 2 handfuls of spinach
- 1 cup of coconut water
- 1/2 avocado
- 1 scoop of Vegan protein powder
- 1-2 other types of superfoods

Creamy Kale Berry

- 1 large handful of blueberries
- 1 large handful of blackberries
- 2 large handfuls of kale
- 1 cup of almond milk
- 1/2 banana
- 1 scoop of vegan protein powder
- 1–2 superfoods.

Cleansing Cucumber Berry

- 1 large handful of strawberries
- 1 large handful of blueberries
- 2 large handfuls of rocket
- 1 cucumber
- 1 cup of aloe vera juice

Berry Butter

- 1 large handful of blueberries
- 1 handful of strawberries,
- 2 handfuls of leafy greens,
- 1 spoonful of peanut butter
- 1 cup of almond milk
- 1/4 cup of gluten-free oats
- 1/2 banana
- 1 scoop of vegan protein powder
- Small spoon of almond butter
- 1–2 superfoods of your choosing

Mangoberry Hempshake

- 1 handful of chopped mangos
- 1 handful of blueberries
- 1 handful of strawberries
- 1 cup of hemp milk

- 2 handfuls of leafy greens
- 1 cup of mineral water
- 1 scoop of Vegan protein powder
- 1–2 superfoods.

Beauty-Boosting Brunch Ideas

During the week, I suggest starting your day with the Elixir of Life Wellness Shot, followed by a **satisfying smoothie** to give your digestion a break from the other meals. However, the following recipes are designed for a tasty brunch style lunch or an indulgent breakfast full of beautifying properties over the weekend, to stay energized all afternoon.

- Scrambled, free-range eggs cooked in coconut oil with chopped avocado and tomatoes. Served with gluten-free toast
- 2 pieces of gluten-free wholegrain toast with a spread of coconut oil and almond butter. Serve with a side of mixed berries
- Gluten-free oatmeal bowl topped with nuts, seeds, apple, cinnamon, and maple syrup. Serve with a side of green salad
- Bowl of homemade muesli made with almonds, goji berries, brazil nuts, walnuts, mixed seeds, blackberries, almond milk and raw honey. Serve with a side of green salad
- 2 slices of gluten-free toast with almond butter spread. Serve with a blueberry, blackberry, spinach, cucumber, and celery smoothie
- Beauty bowl made with gluten-free oats or quinoa, almond milk, and coconut oil, topped with chopped avocado, blueberries, blackberries, nuts, seeds, and pure maple syrup
- Gluten-free pancakes made with gluten-free oats, 1 banana, and egg topped with blueberries, blackberries, and maple syrup
- Free-range eggs with tomatoes, avocados, and peppers

Love-Yourself Lunches

From your door to desk, here are some meals made in just minutes that will energize you all afternoon.

Ashfab Salad Tip: Keep your sumptuous salads in medium-sized mason jars for ready-to-go healthy meals. Start with the dressing and layer your way up. For extra crunch, add extra nuts & seeds.

- **Greek Salad:** Layer from bottom to top with olive oil, balsamic vinegar, diced green peppers, red peppers, cucumber, lettuce, and tomato
- **Chopped Salad:** Layer creamy vegan dressing with diced lettuce, tomatoes, grilled tofu pieces, avocado pieces, and corn
- **Pomegranate Delight:** Layer balsamic vinegar, olive oil, raw honey, spinach, cucumber, pine nuts, green pepper, and pomegranates. Add some goat cheese on top
- **Mango Tango:** Mix olive oil, lemon, black pepper, chopped mango, black beans, avocado, sweet corn, lettuce, red onions
- **Radish Fever:** Layer balsamic vinegar, olive oil, minced garlic, raw honey, sliced radish, chopped lettuce, clementine pieces, shaved almonds, and chopped carrots
- **Spicy shrimp mix:** Layer chili sauce, tamari sauce (gluten-free soy sauce), raw honey, sautéed mushrooms, chopped lettuce, diced avocado, chopped red and green pepper

Ashfab Healthy To-Go Tip: If you are strapped for time and need to grab food on the go, do some research to find healthy, convenient food choices that are free from cow's milk, gluten, and refined sugars.

Look for chunky, dairy and gluten-free soups, savory asian broth soups, sumptuous salads with nuts, seeds, and organic protein, mixed veggies and sushi with little rice, a salmon-style bento box with greens, and gluten-free grain bowls with fresh fruit or veg toppings.

For Asian-style choices, ditch soy sauce and teriyaki; instead, use gluten-free tamari sauce which tastes exactly like soy sauce but contains less salt and no gluten.

Savory Suppers

Warm, savory, light, and satisfying — the perfect way to end the day.

Ashfab Tip: Try to eat at least 3 hours before bedtime; that way, your digestion process will not interrupt your sleep cycles.

- **Sautéed seasonal greens:** choose from courgetti, broccoli, and asparagus. If you wish, add a side of grilled wild salmon.
- **Seared Sea Bass:** add chilli flakes and fresh lemon juice. Serve with seasonal greens
- **southern-style prawns:** add chopped tomatoes, corn, black beans, avocado, and lettuce. Optional: occasionally, it's okay to add grass-fed mince beef or turkey mince rolled in gluten-free or lettuce wraps.
- **Grilled white fish:** serve over cauliflower rice and slightly cooked carrots and corn.
- **Spicy stir fry:** mix with seasonal greens, bean sprouts, and peppers. Cook in coconut oil, and include protein like mushrooms, organic poultry, or side of grilled wild salmon.
- **Plant-based tacos:** fill your gluten-free corn taco shells with avocado, tomatoes, peppers, lettuce, and vegan or grated goat cheese. * Add organic lean meat or fish if you feel you need a protein kick.
- **Gluten-free wholegrain pasta:** top with sautéed mushrooms, kale, broccoli, and grated vegan cheese or pecorino (sheep cheese).
- **Gluten-free wholegrain pasta primavera:** made with organic chopped tomatoes, sea salt, ground black pepper, chilli flakes, garlic, olive oil, and tomato paste. If you feel you need some extra protein, add mushrooms, organic poultry, or tuna chunks.
- **Roasted sweet potato:** mix with butternut squash, and carrots. Top with pomegranates, toasted pine nuts, and a side of grilled tofu steak or a piece of fish.
- **Sautéed seasonal greens:** use kale, peas, and edamame beans, with a side of tofu steak or organic beef.
- **Roasted sweet potato:** top with pomegranates, toasted pine nuts and feta cheese. Serve over wholegrain rice.

Satisfying Snack Ideas

Drink a cold-pressed veggie-based juice with one of the following:

- 1 cup of popcorn
- Some carrot sticks with hummus
- 1 apple with almond butter
- 1-2 plant protein vegan balls
- 1 handful of almonds
- 1 handful of homemade trail mix
- 1 plant-based protein bar that uses dates for sweetener (not cane sugar)
- Plant-based muffin (sugar-free, gluten-free, and dairy-free)

Beauty Food Feasting Overview

Include the age defying trio daily into your wellness regime

Wake Up Energized

Drink an **Elixir of Life Wake-Up Wellness Shot** (ingredients include mineral water, lemon, ginger, turmeric, raw honey, ground black pepper)

Start the Day Right

Drink a homemade, **plant-based green smoothie** with mixed leafy greens, berries, and another fruit, like banana or avocado if you wish. Maximise the nutrients and beauty benefits by adding a scoop of a premium plant-based protein powder from brands like Vega or Garden of Life, a mushroom powder mix, a green powder blend, and other superfoods like maca, chia seeds, then add coconut water or unsweetened vegan milk.

Veggie juice

Include a large glass of fresh, cold-pressed veggie juice with no (except lemon) daily or as often as possible. Homemade or health-store juice is best, preferably organic and locally sourced. Look for raw, fresh, organic or locally sourced if possible if you decide to buy from a shop. This is fab for an afternoon energy boost.

Semi-Fasting is a great way to detox your system daily and help assimilate and absorb vital nutrients. Try not consume your first solid meal until midday, brunch on weekends doesn't really count :-)

Stay Hydrated

Sip on 8–10 glasses of hydrating liquids such as filtered or mineral water (never tap), veggie juices, and herbal tea

Plan for Plants

Plan most of your meals around plants and natural nutrition

Shop Smart

Use the Beauty Food Feasting List and purchase seasonal, organic, locally grown produce. Try new things and be creative in the kitchen

Eliminate Bold-List Foods

Do not consume the foods listed previously in the bold list during the onset of your transformation. After 10 days, save room for occasional treats to celebrate with, **but try not to keep them in the house**

Be a Conscious consumer

Try to shop for organic, locally sourced, seasonal produce whenever possible

Use Smaller Plates

Control your portions by eating from smaller plates. Eat very slowly, take small bites, chew well, and savor the moment

Implement Healthy Swaps

Don't say goodbye to all your favourite foods; instead, try to swap them out for a healthier, plant-based versions. Swap cow's milk for nut milk, carbonara for gluten-free tomato-based spaghetti, deep dish pizza for whole grain sourdough pizza, cappuccino for an almond matcha, and try to choose vegan desserts with less refined sugar

Eat More Fruits & Vegetables

Aim for **7-9 servings** of fruit, especially berries, and vegetables per day, through fresh smoothies, cold-pressed juices, sides, salads, soups, and snacks

Supplementation

Take supplements and superfoods, for optimal cellular health

Focus on feeling great

Before you begin each meal, ask yourself "Is this going to make me feel and look fab? Or drab?" Adopting a beauty food mindset will ultimately lead to better choices

Have a Healthy, Relationship With Food

A nutrition-based mindset will help nourish you for vibrant health, glowing skin, loads of energy, and a sense of inner well-being. Add good foods to crowd out the bad

Release Negative Feelings

Let go of negative feelings toward food, including feeling guilty, counting calories, and strict rules or rigidity. Food is here to fuel us and fill us up. Its purpose is to give us boundless energy, vitality, and inner radiance that will help us shine

Take Baby Steps

Remember, small changes create long-lasting results, so be tedious in your decision-making — it is truly empowering to make healthy choices

Go Natural With a Hint of Naughty

Life is for living, so eat well, but enjoy cake and cocktails as well

Use Your Intuition

An intuitive approach to eating will help you listen to what your body really needs. Ask yourself, "Do I need this, or do I want this?"

Heal Your Gut

If you suffer from tummy troubles or mood disorders and can't ever seem to shift that unwanted belly fat, be mindful of gut irritants like gluten, tap water, processed foods, excess alcohol, and cow's milk not to mention the overuse of antibiotics that strip away healthy bacteria,. These will disrupt your gut health, which can lead to many other health concerns

Go All-In, Then Go 80-20

If you seem to have a long list of health concerns and are overweight, try to follow the plan 100 percent for 8 weeks+ however if you just need a bit of a lifestyle boost than dedicate 10 days and then afterward, try taking the 80-20 approach. Again, it is what you eat most of the time that matters and will either help or harm your health and help fight disease or feed it. So, choose the best natural, fresh ingredients to fill your plate with, and include the **daily age-defying trio** regardless (wellness shot, smoothie, and super juice).

When you complete 10 days of 100 percent commitment, simply switch to the beauty food feasting mindset. Plan your meals around natural nutrition, and eat for your health, well-being and beauty because your skin, cells, and spirit will thank you for it.

"The best project you can ever work on is yourself."

Unknown

PART 2

Feel Fabulous

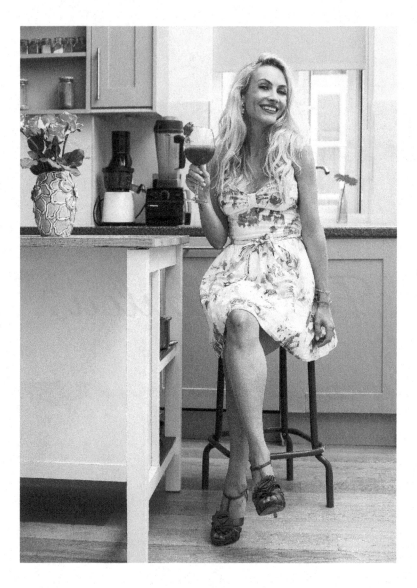

Be such a happy soul,
people crave your high vibes

There is no magic pill to help you feel fabulous; but of course, eating from the beauty food feasting plan will give you tons of energy — not to mention, it will boost your mood, memory, and metabolism while keeping wrinkles, pimples, and rashes at bay.

However, from an emotional point of view, feeling fabulous requires time and effort from ourselves.

Tips & Tools to Feel Fab From the Inside Out

Express Gratitude Daily

First thing in the morning, or right before you go to bed, write down 3–5 things you are grateful for. Appreciate the good, count your blessings, and recognize simple pleasures in life, like having a warm home, hot water, clothes to wear, a beating heart, food on the table, blue skies, blossoming trees, or even rainy days when you stay inside, to be warm and cozy with tea, books, and blankets.

Show your loved ones or someone in your life who may need some extra TLC. It will make them feel good, which in turn will make you feel good. The more gratitude you have in your life, the more joy you will feel, and an abundance of positive things in your life will grow.

Add this habit to your daily routine, whether it's something you do when you go for a walk, get ready for bed, or wake up in the morning. Do whatever suits you best; just be sure to speak it, feel it, act on it, and mean it. By focusing on what we have and being truly grateful for the things around us, happiness will begin to flow. Count your blessings on a daily basis and be grateful for what you have — do not dwell on what you don't have.

A grateful heart will create more abundance in your life. Give thanks, appreciate what you have today, and you will attract more of the same. You'll also feel more positive, hopeful, happy, and optimistic, too.

Begin by appreciating the most basic things in life, like the ability to breathe, the experience of waking up in a cozy bed. Be grateful that you can take a hot shower, listen to the sounds of birds chirping, and that you can always go outside and look up at the blue sky, see or smell the pink flowers blooming. Think about how much nice coffee the barista brightens your morning on your way to work. Focus on your group of friends who support you and have fun with you — you get the idea.

By starting to realize how blessed you are, and seeing what a privilege it is to be alive, to enjoy, love, and laugh, you will finally understand how much you have to be grateful for.

When you begin and end your day with a gratitude for all the little things that there are to be thankful for, it will truly transform your day. You'll go from feeling blah to feeling brilliant.

If I am having a bad day or feeling a little off, I take some time to meditate and think of things I'm grateful for. When you adopt and develop an attitude of gratitude, it will bring not only powerful and positive emotions to your sense of well-being, but you will also strengthen your immune system, have more clarity in life, and elevate your mood. Make an effort to cultivate a grateful heart, and you will naturally increase love, joy, hope, and inner peace on a daily basis.

> **"A grateful, loving, kind heart is the true gateway to joy and abundance."**
>
> **—Ashley Siedentopf**

Positive Vibes

Struggles and stress from relationships, money, work, and illness can take a toll on your health and mood. Even if you're experiencing tough times, you've got to stay as positive and upbeat as you can. What you focus on in life expands, so if something goes wrong, do not keep complaining, obsessing, or thinking about it, otherwise the situation will just feel and possibly become worse.

Be strong, and turn any negative thoughts, actions, or comments into happier ones, even in the darkest times. Being positive doesn't mean life is always smooth-sailing; however, positive people have real-life problems that make them upset and angry too — but they practice resilience. They fight for what they believe in.

It's not about having your head in the clouds and thinking everything is just perfect, and it's no good to ignore the real issues when life gets tough.

However, it is vital to hold yourself accountable for your emotional state and to be aware of your thoughts and feelings. It is not about denying what is going on or suppressing emotions either — this will negatively impact your mental and physical health.

The best approach to adopting a positive mindset through tough times is to recognise negative thoughts and actively transform them into positive ones as often as you can. This will have a profound effect on your health and well-being. Call a friend you know you can confide in, and if they're okay with it, have a speech-vomit session, as I call it. Just vent, get it off your chest, breathe, and move on.

If you are constantly complaining, and seeing situations as the worst case scenarios, well, that's exactly the energy you are going to get back! Even when life is a little grey and not how you wish it was, you just need to train your brain to be more optimistic. Choose to look on the bright side of life, look forward to wonderful new adventures and focus on feeling things that make you feel good.

When you notice yourself having a negative thought, bad day, or low mood, stop whatever you are doing, and think of three positive thoughts, make a gratitude list, go get some fresh air, get out in nature, go for a walk, or call a friend — and watch your mood go from blah to brilliant in minutes.

There are times when we will go through some really tough moments, lose loved ones, have a bad breakup, feel physically exhausted, or just simply suffer. Yes, life can totally be complicated, but when you are positive, you look for solutions and find the best choice for the situation, whatever it may be. And yes, it's also okay to not be okay sometimes; just be sure to train your brain to stay optimistic, resilient, and positive as much as you can. After a while, your way of thinking, speaking, and talking will become more positive. Being a positive person can truly transform your outlook on life and change how you react and respond to events and situations. Being positive makes you more resilient to stress and struggles! You have the power to be positive every day, and when you are having a negative moment, then think of something that you appreciate at that moment, that alone will shift your mindset instantly.

A positive mindset is a very important part of the fab formula. It takes time, and effort, to rock a positive attitude, but do it anyway! Choose to be positive, act positive, think positive, live positive, spread positive vibes, and have positive expectations! Happiness, a positive attitude, and good energy are contagious, so it's important to maintain happy, high vibes as much as you can because they will boomerang right back to you.

The more you make an effort to be positive in your life, the more you will generate feelings of happiness and well-being, making you glow and radiate positivity from within — and that is the sort of energy people want to be around.

High Vibe Living

When you truly begin to pay attention to your vibes, you will shift your energy from within, strengthen your personal power, and ultimately, get positive vibes in return. I am a firm believer in the idea that "the universe serves what you deserve" for the most part.

There are so many possible positive and negative emotions and feelings that we can experience daily. In order for you to live with and emit elevated vibes and attract more awesomeness and goodness in your life, it is important to stay in the high vibe range.

"High vibes" include:

- positive outlook
- hope
- faith
- belief in the unknown
- enthusiasm
- appreciation
- joy
- love
- kindness
- creativity
- knowledge
- compassion
- passion
- empowerment

"Low vibes" are based on:

- fear
- anger
- sadness
- depression
- criticism
- resentment
- rigidness
- guilt
- jealousy
- judgment
- insecurity
- worry
- pessimism
- boredom
- doubt
- blame

As you begin to shift your mindset to focus on high vibe living, pay attention when low vibes are dominating your thought processes and mental patterns, so you can actively change them. Strengthening your mind to stay in the high-vibes zone, takes practice; however, with time, self-awareness, and dedication, you will soon realize it is only you who creates both good and bad vibes from within.

Do not let external factors get the best of you. If you are struggling currently, try being hopeful or having faith in the future, and focus on other good things. Either way, program your mind to focus on high vibe living. Again, positive vibes will boomerang back to you — I can promise you that. So, own your vibes, and be that person you would want to spend time with.

Love Thyself

Learning to love yourself, truly, and wholeheartedly takes practice, commitment, and dedication. It is extremely important to be kind and compassionate to yourself, and to embrace who you are. When you love yourself, your true spirit shines bright from within.

Those who love themselves are more tuned into their thoughts and feelings rather than the negative noise that the outside world feeds us. Remember: no pill, potion, or person can make us feel loved. Truly, you must fall in love with yourself first. Forget focusing on your flaws. Embrace your qualities and remind yourself how fabulous you are.

If you struggle with low self-esteem or find it difficult to practice self-love, start today. Make a commitment to love yourself. Self-love is kind and empathetic; it is knowing who you are and what you like and don't like. Self-love is not selfish — it is selfless. It's paying attention to your qualities and attributes and sharing them with the world. It is recognising your flaws, but forgiving yourself since no one is perfect. It's about owning your weaknesses and working on them. Be kind to yourself, speak to yourself with kind words, as if you were speaking to your friend, quiet that negative self talk in your head, this is all just complete nonsense anyways, simply just be you, love yourself, and remember you are a beautiful soul just the way you are.

Ditch the Compare-and-Despair Fixation.

Do not get fixated on other peoples picture-perfect lives, looks and journeys. Each and every one of us is beautiful in our own way, and when we love ourselves whole-heartedly, it is much easier to freely share the love, compassion and compliments to others around us. Do not compare where you are in life to where someone else is. Be patient with yourself, focus on your dreams and desires, and remember you can do anything you put your mind too. Resentment and jealousy do not serve us in any way, shape, or form. Instead, they make it much more difficult for us to become truly radiant souls.

So, my darling, make it a priority to fall in love with yourself from this day forward. If you are lacking in the self-love department, set aside 15 minutes daily for 21 days, and without stopping, list all your achievements and things that make you wonderful. This can be as simple as a, "I am a loyal friend," or, "I make the best banana bread," or "I am a loving daughter," "I make people laugh," "I am a good listener," and so on.

By creating a list of all the things that make you unique, fabulous, and exceptional, you will greatly boost your inner beauty.

By becoming aware of all the fab things about you, and expressing yourself openly and honestly, you will give off a magnetic vibe and attract all kinds of love from different directions. Loving thyself is the key to true inner peace and fulfilment. Forget perfection. Stop comparing yourself to others. Be you. Love you. Embrace you. And just be yourself.

**"Your energy does all the talking and vibes say it all....
good or bad ones"**

Ashley Siedentopf

Be Kind

Humility, kindness, and compassion for others are what will elevate your karmic energy. What you put out and give out will only come back to you. So, sending out good vibes to others, being empathetic, staying humble, and having kind thoughts will only add goodness to your life.

If you are sincere, genuine, and generous with your thoughts and attitude, you will receive this kind of energy in return from your friends, family, partners, co-workers or random acts of kindness. When you are stingy with your thoughts, resentful, jealous, judgmental and inconsiderate of others, you will experience more negativity in your life.

So, throw kindness around like colourful confetti and watch it grow your spirit and strengthen your soul. When you combine your joy with gratitude and a kind heart, you will have a real magnetic force that will keep attracting abundance, positive vibes, and beautiful experiences.

**"Kindness creates karma too. So, think kind thoughts,
speak kind words, do kind deeds, and karma will bite
you on the ass with kindness."**

Unknown

Affirm Awesome Thoughts

The power of affirmations is life changing. By affirming your thoughts, you instantly shift your mindset to believing what you wish will happen is already happening. If you want to lose weight, tell yourself, "I am strong, slim, and healthy." If you want to thrive in your career, remind yourself, "I am successful." If you need a confidence boost, remind yourself how beautiful, amazing, and talented you are. Affirm what you want, and say it from the heart often.

This may all sound a little hokey, but take this, for example. In 2013, I remember writing down things that I wanted, including an amazing wedding in Ibiza, a career doing what I love, and an adorable puppy. So I wrote in my journal, "I am designing my dream job. I have a beautiful, whimsical wedding in Ibiza. And I have the perfect puppy."

A couple years later, I quit my job, went back to nutrition school, launched a health and beauty blog, wrote an eBook, started my own cooking channel, got the most adorable pug in the world, and pulled of an amazing, memorable wedding in Ibiza with all of our nearest, dearest and loved ones.

Being a "goal digger," I always try to evolve, reinvent myself, reach for the stars, and become the best version of me. As my own boss, I do experience challenges, tough times, and bad days; however, positive affirmations remind me of why I do what I do. They serve as an instant mood booster.

Write your daily affirmations in a place where you can see them constantly. Repeat these affirmations regularly throughout the day. Using the power of affirmations regularly will help make your dreams come true. It may seem a little out of this world to those of you not familiar with the concept, but trust me, it works! I believe where I am today in life today comes down to a combo of daily meditation, daily affirmations, self-love, supportive friends and family, and staying as optimistic and positive as I can even during tough times.

I still have a long way to go in pursuing my goals, but either way, I was working in the corporate world, unfulfilled, but decently paid, and learned a lot. When I finally built up the courage to quit and go to nutrition school,

I freed myself. I am still "Ash," but I am more self-aware, present, and conscious however a huge goofball, fun-loving, free spirit at heart.

I use affirmations every day which are simply a positive pre tense phase, they are a great natural mood booster and reminder to live life fully, never give up on your dreams, believe in yourself completely, and keep going during darker times.

The attention you give to something is what will flourish, good or bad, so it really is paramount to associate positive emotions with your affirmations. You must feel, act, and speak about what you want.

Favourite Daily Affirmations

- "Having mega confidence, a clear vision, compassion, and creativity will bring me great rewards."
- "I am amazing, beautiful, intelligent, whole, and loving."
- "I am grateful for the abundance of health, beauty, and love in my life."
- "I attract what I want easily and freely. I focus on positivity, abundance, and excellence. Everything I do is filled with joy, love, and blessings."
- "I am living the life of my dreams today."
- "I am moving closer toward my goals every single day."
- "I believe in myself, and I am unstoppable."
- "Staying on the path of beauty, love, peace, joy, and appreciation brings me true happiness and abundance."
- "I am worthy of receiving gifts of joy, peace, and prosperity"
- "I am successful."
- "I am a wonderful mother."

"Optimism is a happiness magnet. If you stay positive, good things and good people will be drawn to you."

—Mary Lou Retton

Accept the Past and Let Go

Throughout life, I have gone through some bumps and bruises along the way, but with each mistake and struggle came a lesson. I learned that whatever adversity we are facing, we must accept it and feel our emotions, even if it hurts.

This includes allowing ourselves to feel grief, loss, sickness, and sadness. If we deny reality and never come to terms with our inner experience, we become mentally unhealthy. Holding feelings and thoughts inside, repressing experiences, and denying or escaping reality have very negative effects on our emotional, mental, and spiritual health in the long run.

Holding in feelings and emotions is extremely unhealthy. Even if it is extremely difficult, it is important to meet with friends who you can be open with, call a therapist for professional guidance, grab a journal and do daily mind dumps to get it out on paper — anything! If you have deep dark secrets or unresolved issues with family and friends, decide right here and now that you are going to deal with it. If you do, your mental health and happiness will thank you big time.

Once you have made it to the other side, you will feel like you are dropping a boulder you have been dragging along. Keeping things bottled up is so bad for our inner and outer health. It eats away at us, causing stress, anxiety, and worse, depression.

Be brave and make an effort to heal old wounds, come to terms with them, get the support you need, and get it out in the open. Secondly, when things arise that are not so easy keep a strong mindset. Accept that it's okay to not be okay, and that feeling pain is a part of life. Allow yourself to feel all emotions that you go through, and then put them in a balloon and let them go into the air. Once you do, you'll finally be able to relax, breathing in fresh, crisp air and exhaling to release every ounce of tension.

Putting on a brave face and making it seem like everything is okay when it's not is actually not very brave. Facing struggles and tough times takes far more courage and bravery, and in the end, you will feel lighter, brighter, and better for it. Face hardship, feel it, accept it, and let it go. Get back on that horse and look forward to it!

During the latter half of 2017, while I was writing this book, I had a miscarriage at almost 10 weeks, which left me pretty weak emotionally, mentally, and physically. It took several months for me to finally feel like myself again, and it also affected my thyroid, which left me weak and lethargic. And then, right before Christmas, I was given news that no one ever wants to hear: my husbands father, an amazing human that I had the privilege to know for seven years, had committed suicide. It was a complete shock, and it happened right before the holidays.

Experiencing those two losses within six months of each other was pretty painful to say the least. I was deeply affected by the suicide emotionally; however, I found out I was pregnant right after the holidays, and it felt like an absolute miracle, a gift from god. We were now given another life to nourish, nurture, and love, so the new year started off in deep grief, many tears, and heartache, as well, an intense maternal need to protect the little baby growing inside me. I hoped, prayed, and had faith that I would not go through the pain of miscarriage again.

The point is, even though my miscarriage & the sudden death took a huge toll on me, I had to simply put health first. I decided to slow down, focus on my family, and have faith that one day, I would have a healthy baby. This shift in my mindset helped me significantly, because I let go of expectations of myself and my future.

Don't get me wrong, there are still many sad moments that come up, especially since my daughter will never know her grandfather, even though he would have made an amazing one. When we lose loved ones, it is best to speak about them, remember them, celebrate them, and to never forget all the goodness they gave while they were here on earth. And most of all, it is important to be grateful for all the good memories we had with them.

"Don't deny your pains or sorrows. They are gifts that help you find courage to gain wisdom and healing, for wholeness and peace"

—Elaine Mary Collins

Bye bye negativity

Negative emotions and low-vibe mental chatter in your head can wreak havoc on your inner health and beauty. Fear, anger, guilt, insecurity, jealousy, worry, doubt, lack of self-worth, moodiness, anxiety, resentment, judgment, criticism, and irritability, eat away at our emotional, mental, spiritual, and physical health. As you begin to pay more attention to your inside and outside health, you need to learn to zap those negative thoughts, emotions, and feelings before they fester in your mind.

An exercise that will help you do this is to practice visualisation every time you shower. As you cleanse your body, think of all your bad vibes and emotions, such as work stress, waking up feeling agitated, or financial worry, and imagine all your negativity being rinsed away and circling down the drain. It's like spring-cleaning your mind daily. Since thoughts are just in our mind, it's important to recognize them, understand that it's okay to not be okay, be mindful of the moment, and let them go if they do not serve us. Learning to release negative vibes, feelings, and emotions is key to getting through hardship and becoming a healthier, happier person.

Hearing, speaking, and reading negative things has a huge impact on your emotional and mental health. What you decide to listen to can lift you up or lower your sense of peace, joy, and happiness. Be careful about what you choose to fill your mind, body, and soul with. Ditch negative thoughts, emotions, pressures and opinions.

Release negativity and replace it with positive emotions, thoughts, words and affirmations as much as you can. This will open the gateway to abundance, joy, accomplishment, and peace. Negative thoughts, beliefs, and limitations will sabotage your success in all areas of your life, such as your career, finances, relationships, choices, habits, and creativity. Become more aware of your thoughts and negative thinking patterns.

Even when life seems like you're in the deep end due to the loss of loved one, financial struggles, or illness, you must try to prevail, and look at the bigger picture. Work through your struggles one day at a time, and have hope and faith that in the future, you will be okay again. After all, "This too shall pass." Use this mantra when you are suffering to remind yourself that you'll feel better eventually.

As much as I don't glorify or agree with "dieting" or calorie-counting, I highly recommend going on a mental diet that cuts out negativity and complaining — doing so will truly make life seem so much more precious.

Fab Friends and Family

The people in your life have a huge effect on your energy, decisions, memories, and experiences. Surround yourself with people who are uplifting, nurturing, supportive, genuine, kind, sincere, positive, loving, and wholesome. These relationships will lift you up, inspire you, and bring out the best in you. Real friends are good listeners, are always there for you, and feel truly excited about your success or good things that happen to you, and of course there for tough times, which can strike at any point. These people are what I call the radiators.

The drains, however, are the Debbie Downers, the Moaning Minnies, or the Negative Nancys. They complain all the time, have a negative vibe, are pessimistic, resentful and jealous, sometimes without you even noticing, and they don't bring much value to your life. They give advice based only on their own life, tell white lies, never evolve, and have constant problems in their life; even if you give them advice often, they just go in circles (which I call ask-holes).

If you end up feeling tired, frazzled, drained, or annoyed after you see or speak to these people, it is a sign to keep your distance. Family is family, but when it comes to toxic people, you must set the boundaries that you need, whether that means limiting how often you see them or cutting them out altogether. You have a life too, and sometimes you need to be self-centered to keep your life in balance to stay on top of things.

You may have many close friends who have always been there for you during difficult times; however, can you also ask yourself, are they also your biggest supporters and fans when things are going great? The answer may surprise you. Most of us have one or two friends who will help you when things go wrong, but at the same time, they don't have your back when life is going great and things are flowing, happening, and evolving.

Your true friends will be so happy for you in both good and bad times. They'll have your back in awesome moments and darker times! Surround yourself with people who are uplifting, make you laugh, let you be you, and bring out the best in you — not the stress in you!

Adjust Your Mindset

Although my book contains a wealth of tips, tricks, and tools that I use for living a healthy lifestyle, one thing I know for sure is what has been paramount to my healing journey is my mindset. I'm not just talking about the positive, optimistic, "look at the bright side" way of thinking; it's more than that. I never let myself play the victim, and when I feel sick, even when I was prescribed a daunting list of medications while being bed-bound, or going through some sort of serious struggle, I make sure I don't act or think like I'm sick or swimming in struggle. I never play the "poor me" role or ask for a pity party.

Instead, I try to shift my mindset and say, "Ash, get back on the horse and move forward." If you are going through some type of health imbalance, relationship issue, financial constraints, or other struggles, feeling sorry for yourself does you no justice. If you have been feeling low, lethargic towards life, or just generally not living fully, you must take the reins and know that you are responsible for your life story. Sure, you cannot control external factors that may have taken place; however, you can control your mindset, your responses to it, and how you live in the present. So make your mindset one that is strong, resilient, and takes no B.S from life itself.

"Never let a bad day, make you feel you have a bad life"

Unknown

Meditate

Back in the day, I thought meditation, mantras, and mindfulness were just for full-time yogis, but once I started to implement more spirituality into my lifestyle, everything changed for the better. Today I am an advocate for positive living, grateful thinking, healthy eating, daily exercising, and compassionate loving. The more I tapped into my spiritual side, the more I felt fab and full of life, despite hurdles and hard times.

Feeling a little lost and don't know where to start? Begin by reading books on gratitude, positivity, self-discovery, and spirituality. Incorporate yoga (a form of meditation) into your exercise routine, and download a guided meditation app to follow. I now meditate once a day for 20 minutes. By adding meditation to your daily wellness regime you will be more mindful of your choices, thoughts and actions in life, feel more grounded, have better concentration and ability to stay focused during work, be less anxious during stressful situations, and have a positive and optimistic attitude towards today and the future. You'll also cultivate a sense of inner peace, balance, and harmony form within.

Other fab benefits of meditation include improved sleep, stronger immune system, boosted metabolism, stronger connection to others, and deep appreciation for life. It also increases creativity and serotonin levels, as well as increased self-actualization & compassion. Meditation encourages peace of mind and happiness and keeps things in perspective.

By making meditation a part of your daily health regime, you will feel a big difference in your sense of well-being. As you meditate more often, you will begin to feel more expansive, connected to others, conscious of your thoughts and feelings, as well as a clear sense of who you truly are and what brings you joy.

Check out guided meditation websites or download meditation apps. If you can, wake up a little earlier so that you can start your day stress-free with a feeling of clarity contentment, and peace of mind. If you can do one meditation session before bed, you'll doze off with good thoughts in your subconscious mind.

Beauty Sleep

The amount and quality of your sleep has a huge impact on the health of your body and skin. Anything under a solid 7 hours can cause immediate signs of aging including puffy eyes, prominent wrinkles, and acne, not to mention you'll be more prone to colds, flus, and infections. Lack of sleep also makes you way more cranky, short-tempered, and increases the likelihood that you'll reach for a starchy foods in the morning. This is because sleep deprivation directly impacts sugar and carbohydrate cravings.

Sleeping for less than 7 hours will hinder your health, well-being, and beauty in the long run. In fact, when I am sleep deprived, I can feel signs right away —I feel totally zombie-like and irritable and look 10 years older. Strive for 8–9 hours of uninterrupted sleep, this will have a positive impact on your health, well-being and beauty.

A nighttime ritual is my favourite way to ensure I get those ZZZs. One hour before bed, switch off your phone, TV, and other screens. Take a hot bath with Epsom salt to relax and soothe your muscles. If you don't have a tub, do a dry-brush body scrub with salt. Try using magnesium nighttime spray to naturally relax and calm your mind, drop some lavender essential oils on your palms, and breathe three times, sip soothing bedtime tea, like chamomile and lavender. Jot down some notes in your journal including thoughts of the day, what went well, a gratitude list, and anything else on your mind. Read something inspirational for at least 20 minutes before sleeping to leave your subconscious mind with uplifting thoughts.

Commit to getting 8–9 hours of sleep during the week to receive the benefits of a full night's sleep. Beauty sleep boosts energy levels and brain power, combats stress, curbs cravings, and keeps you looking beautiful all day, every day. (This obviously does not apply to new mamas. If you've just had a baby, be gentle with yourself and do your best to get some rest, and throw out any guilt if you need to lay down when your baby does. My daughter is close to 16 months and still doesn't always sleep solid, so if I am getting broken sleep, I will rest for a disco nap the following day)

Bedtime Routine Checklist

Supplies include:

- Magnesium spray
- Soothing Bedtime tea
- Lavender essential oils
- Journal
- Inspirational reading material and a selections of crystals next to my bed or under my pillow
- A couple of drops of cbd oil by Pure hemp plus

Give yourself a good hour before you intend to fall asleep so you have time for your bedtime routine, and put away the phone. If you come home late, simply cleanse your skin and go to bed, However, on the nights where you're in bed before midnight, like Cinderella, a bedtime routine is the perfect way to close the day. If you have kids, put them to bed at the same time every night so you can follow your routine and have some "me" time. Happy mama, happy kids. ;-)

Journaling

Going through some stress at home or work? Is there something that is bothering you currently? Perhaps you have an idea for a business, but you feel a bit anxious about it, or maybe your mind is racing and thinking about the million things you need to do.

Bottling emotions and feelings is extremely unhealthy for inner health, especially before sleep time. Writing your thoughts and emotions out in a journal before bed is a great way to get out all the worries. It simply helps you get it all off your chest and see the clearer picture. There's no one to judge you — it's just you and your trust notepad. Get it all out and move on.

When I started journaling every night before bed, I found that I fell asleep more easily and woke up feeling happier and worry-free. I also write down five things that went well in my day and five things I am grateful for, so I always fall asleep with a smile.

Journaling doesn't just have to be just writing about worries and stress; it can be about dreams, and inspiration and it doesn't have to have a structure or a real purpose, either. It's just a meditative practice to help you clear your mind and process your thoughts. Sit for a few minutes every day and write out anything that comes to your mind, good, bad, happy, or sad. Write without stopping and don't worry about your spelling or grammar. This is so great for your soul and spirit because it is also activating your fifth Chakra, which is in your throat and is all about speaking the truth, being bold, expressing confidence, and simply being true to yourself. Go get yourself a pretty journal and do a daily mind dump.

Ashfab Feel-Good Tip: keep a cute journal and pen next to your bed where you can see it. Once you get in bed, sit and write for just a few minutes, jotting down anything that comes to your mind for a better sleep.

Inhale Essential Oils

Essential oils are organic compounds extracted from plants with tremendous healing properties that help to boost physical, mental, emotional and spiritual health. You can use essential oils by aromatic diffusion, topical application, and dietary consumption. You will enhance your health and well-being by adding different types of organic botanical drops to your wellness regime.

I started using essential oils during the spring of 2017, and got totally hooked. Living in a fast-paced city like London, where it's all go-go-go, can be slightly stressful (no matter how zenned out you are). That's why I like to mix up scents that are uplifting, balancing, calming, and soothing throughout the day.

First thing in the morning, I use a citrus scent like orange or grapefruit for energizing, invigorating, happiness-promoting vibes, and uplifting benefits. After lunch I rub a few drops of a balance-themed mix I made from geranium and Ylang Ylang into my palms. This is a very grounding blend, and it promotes a sense of calmness and evokes feelings of tranquility and balance. Sometimes, I prefer to use a potent peppermint blend to give me an afternoon kick and help me focus and concentrate instead.

Lastly after a nice Epsom salt soak, I use a lavender blend before bedtime. The scent is so soothing, relaxing, and helps promote a peaceful sleep as well as reduces any anxiety or tension.

Experiment and play around with the beautiful scents. Look for premium organic brands, and choose whatever you like best, as there are many different scents that give different benefits.

Practice Yoga

I really got into yoga around six years ago and love to mix it up with different styles like ashtanga, hot, vinyasa, yin and restorative yoga around. As I have deepened my practice on the mat, I have also strengthened my mind, body, soul, and spirit at the same time. Yoga is not just about holding dynamic poses; it combines breathing, moving, and meditating into one practice, so it has a profound effect on your mental, physical, emotional, and spiritual health.

No one is ever too young or too old to reap the health benefits of yoga, as there are modifications for every fitness level. There are several types of yoga to choose from, so find the one that is best suited to your needs and goals. Physically speaking, yoga creates a toned, flexible, and strong body, and it also improves energy and vitality, helping you maintain a balanced metabolism. Mentally speaking, yoga helps you relax and let go of the stresses of life, and it encourages positive thoughts and self-acceptance. And lastly, spiritually speaking, it builds awareness of your body, your feelings, the world around you, the needs of others, and much more.

I highly recommend yoga for those who suffer from any stress, anxiety or depression, as it really does help calm the mind. By making yoga an important part of your health and wellness regime you will find inner peace from within (without having to fly to an exotic beach), and you will improve your flexibility and relieve stress (stress can speed up the signs of ageing and make you sick).

By practicing yoga often with different dynamic classes, you can expect to have a long, lean, sculpted physique. Yoga is a total body workout, for your mind, body and spirit, so I say Namaste to that!

> **"Wellness is the state of being in fab physical, mental, and spiritual health. It is that beautiful balance between body, mind, and spirit."**
>
> **—Ashley Siedentopf**

Stay Mentally Motivated

Maintaining motivation during your new path to vibrant health, natural beauty, and inner well-being requires discipline, dedication, and doing something every day to bring you closer to your goals.

Motivation is the force that guides our behaviours to get results. Believing and visualizing how you want to look and feel means you're already halfway there, so set a goal to visualize everything you want down to the last detail!

See it, feel it, eat it, and breath it. When you visualize and focus on the outcome, you will automatically feel more excited and energized to do whatever it is you need to do. While you're on this path to fabulosity, implement the 3 Ps and stay Positive, Patient, and Persistent. Adopt an upbeat, grateful, positive attitude, and do not compare yourself to others. The comparison and despair can really bring you down, leave you feeling hopeless. Being motivated takes daily action, tenacity, and a deep level of focus. It means taking small steps toward your goal so that you can succeed.

Follow Your Joy

No matter where you are in your life at this time, your ultimate goal and highest purpose should be to feel joyful and happy. You may have a wardrobe full of expensive handbags and designer heels; however, "things" really only give you instant gratification — and I say that as someone who thoroughly enjoys swiping that credit card and taking home a sexy pair of shoes or a new gorgeous new jumpsuit, — but it is not the material things that truly bring us a deep sense of joy, contentment, and true happiness.

There are millions of sites and books on how to be happy and joyful, but it truly comes down to making a simple decision to be happy. If you're reading this now and in a bit of a funk or going through a tough time, you need to focus on things and activities that bring you joy, light you up and make you happy.

Take some alone time, turn your phone off for a weekend, and write a list of things that you love doing. For me, it would be cooking, going to the local market on a saturday, diving into a good book, flipping through some fashion magazines, taking bubble baths, getting a massage, spending time in nature, coloring, having a girls' night out, meeting for lunch with a good friend, hanging with my hubby, cooking for loved ones, taking a yoga class, or going for a walk in nature. Although these examples may sound quite basic, they really do make me feel happy and content.

After my miscarriage summer 2017, something that is common for many women but not openly talked about, I felt so sad, heartbroken, weak, tired, and just generally low. After reading some stories of other mums who went through something similar, I thought to myself after a week of being pretty much on bedrest, "Ash, it is up to you to get out of this funk, no one else. You need to accept what happened, not blame yourself, and not feel ashamed, or ask 'why?' Just get back on the horse, move forward, accept what is, have faith in what will be, and focus on feeling good, slowing down, healing mentally and emotionally, believing, trusting and letting go."

I've always been a very happy-go-lucky, optimistic, positive kind of girl, no matter what life threw at me. But after this experience, I never wanted to feel so low again. No, it wasn't easy, but like I said, no magic pill, potion, or possession can lift you up. It is all about your mindset: you have to choose to be happy and focus on the things that bring you joy.

In case you've forgotten what it feels like, joy is that feeling of your heart singing, feeling good, staying present, not dwelling on the past, or fretting over the future, but being here, right now, and smiling from the inside out. Feeling joyful and happy is your birthright, so wherever you are in life, choose joy to be your highest purpose and main goal, and whatever it is that makes you feel joyful, do more of that!

Simmer That Stress

Modern day living, work, family, financial constraints, deadlines, to-do lists, or simply the demands of life itself can bring up all sorts of strain, struggle, and pressure from within. A small amount of stress obviously is normal and somewhat "healthy"; however, when you let stress eat you up inside and take over your mind, body, and spirit, it eventually will develop into chronic stress, which causes all sorts of other health struggles; not to mention, it accelerates aging and can leads to a lifestyle related illness and saggy skin. Stress is always going to pop up in your life; however, you can really help the situation by switching your mindset.

As you gain a better sense of awareness around you with your thoughts, actions, and feelings, ask yourself: "Am I causing the stress, by being dramatic, difficult and complex, or am I reacting to it by moaning, being negative, and only making matters worse by harping and dwelling? Or am I searching for a solution, who tries to take a step back, knows that everything will be okay, stays calm, doesn't think of the worst-case scenario, and is cool as a cucumber even if life has just fallen into a million pieces?" When things are a bit more stressful, try to focus on solutions the right way, not worst-case scenarios.

Are you the creator, reactor, or problem-solver? Okay, I get it if it's that time of the month; hormones can really make situations worse, but generally speaking, try to avoid creating drama or reacting irrationally. Instead, go for a walk, do a meditation session, book a yoga class or call a bestie and vent it out.

Stress is a part of life; however, as you only get to live on this earth once, the best thing you can do for your health, well-being, and beauty is to be a stress problem-solver, rather than being a creator or reactor. By trying to remain calm when there is a storm brewing, you will benefit in your relationships, work, career, and family life; plus, you will age much better, as stress literally is one of the biggest contributors to both belly fat, under eye bags, and wrinkles. When you make yoga and meditation a part of your lifestyle, you will naturally reduce levels and also become more resilient to adversity in the process.

> **"Relationship status: committed to inner peace, self-love, growth, and gratitude."**
>
> **Unknown**

Lighten Up & Laugh

Laughing is truly an amazing way to naturally boost your health and sense of well-being. One of the best feelings in the world is that knee-slapping, LMAO (laughing my a$$ off) kind of giggle with loved ones.

The health benefits of having a sense of humour and laughing are incredible. Laughter strengthens your immune system, boosts and elevates your mood, helps diminish pain from the endorphins, lowers blood pressure, strengthens resilience towards struggles, protects you from the damaging effects of stress, eases anxiety, and helps you feel more joyful and creative in life. So try to spend time with those who are fun and playful, don't take life so seriously, so try to have a sense of humor and be someone who can easily laugh at yourself.

For a healthy social hangout, go out for a bite to eat and let your hair down, or watch a funny movie or TV series with your family and friends. Find something entertaining and light-hearted. Humor is good for your mental health and will help you have a more positive attitude and optimistic outlook in difficult situations because it will give you a boost and help you feel better. Actually my best memories are always the ones that are so spontaneous and random, and I look back at them and still laugh out loud.

"A day without laughter is a day wasted."

—Unknown

Do All With Love

Love is everything; love is what makes the world go 'round; love is what lights us up; love is in our nature. From this day forward, whatever you are doing at any given moment, whether it be calling your mum, writing an essay, building a new shelf, taking a yoga class, creating a piece of art, cooking, or writing an email, be fully present. Speak and think with love. Be in each moment with as much love as you can, even if it is not something you are keen on doing. Switching your mindset to love rather than fear will make whatever you are doing much more pleasant and happy.

Try Holistic Therapies

As a wellness enthusiast and holistic health advocate, I will forever be on this journey to improving my life and sharing it with those around me. I am on a mission to eat and feel my best today and every day, and to look my best too. Feeling well is not just about the food we put in our mouth or the vigorous workouts at the gym; feeling balanced, beautiful, happy, and healthy is a whole formula, and sometimes, struggles, and stress can take over, causing life to not-so smooth sailing.

Indulging in a holistic treatment or two could be the perfect answer to help you boost your overall sense of well-being and to provide your body and mind with self-care.

Therapies like acupuncture, reiki and deep tissue massages are incredibly beneficial and are my go-to's for extra support on my wellness journey. All three give you different benefits. For example, deep tissue massages melt away stress and release tensions; stress in my eyes is as dangerous as unhealthy food. It really is a silent killer, as it accelerates ageing, makes you feel frazzled and unfeminine, contribute to poor eating and lifestyle habits, zaps energy, and can cause a ray of other chronic health problems. So instead of cocktail night with your girls, maybe a mega-pampering session for yourself every so often would benefit you even more.

When you check in at an acupuncture center, the doctor usually checks your tongue and your pulse rate. After this assessment, he will treat and locate the meridians that need more attention. Acupuncture targets specific points of the body that need some extra attention, as well as areas that feel slightly off. It can effectively help balance that specific area out. I have been having acupuncture done weekly to help rejuvenate my fertility after my miscarriage and have seen a huge improvement in my energy levels.

I had my first reiki session in autumn of 2017, and I now have monthly sessions with a healer. It is such a magical experience! Not only is each session different, it varies for each person. It helps you feel very relaxed and experience different types of sensations that promote peace, harmony, and balance within you. This enables you to handle and cope with stress and tough times much more easily. Reiki targets your physical, mental, emotional, and spiritual health, enhancing all areas of your life to strengthen your inner and outer being.

Open and Aligned Chakras

Firstly, if you are new to the term chakras, here's a brief overview: chakras are energy centers within your body and around your aura. The human body contains three systems: physical, emotional, and energetic life. Your chakra system exists in the energetic body. There are seven chakras from the base of your spine all the way up to the crown of your head. These are the seven main energy centers of your body.

Each chakra causes a positive effect when it is open and a negative effect if it is closed. The chakras exude strong life force energy throughout the body. They truly act as windows to our inner selves, connecting physical, mental, emotional, and spiritual health together. Think of them as portals to your inner and outer world.

I became really interested in the power of chakras from my reiki sessions due to the fact that my healer was able to detect which chakras were open, aligned and activated, and which ones were blocked and imbalanced. I found this absolutely fascinating.

For example, one of the first times I went for reiki, my root chakra was blocked, and I had a lot of sensations around my knees, which stems from the feeling of instability, not feeling grounded, belonging, secure or safe. And it was true! I was juggling quite a few things in terms of my work. Although I always have big dreams, I doubted myself many times and was unsure where I was headed and how I was going to get there, so fear would come up, in terms of financial constraints or "what if's?"

When your chakras are aligned, open, and activated, you will feel amazing, high-energy, happy, empowered and strong in all areas of your life.

The best way to boost your chakra system is to visualize the colour of each chakra while affirming the suggested phrases to help open and activate them. For extra support to keep your chakras open, aligned and balanced, try regular reiki sessions, affirmations and daily chakra healing meditations found on apps like Insight Timer.

Balance Your Chakras and become the best version of yourself.

Chakra 1: Root

Chakra 1 is located at the base of your spine, near your tailbone. It's colour is red, and it represents the foundation and feeling of being grounded, rooted, and taking care of your basic needs. When it is **in balance**, you will feel secure, and experience a sense of belonging, high energy, and healthy body awareness.

Signs & Symptoms of Imbalanced Root Chakra

- Fear
- Insecurity
- Lack of Self-Belief

- Low Self-Esteem
- Depression
- Anxiety
- Addictive behaviour

Visualize red at the base of the spine and affirm the following:

- I am abundant in every area in my life
- I am confident
- I have everything I need
- I belong and I am worthy of greatness
- I release the past
- Mother earth always supports me

Chakra 2: Sacral

The sacral chakra is orange and located below your belly button. When activated and open, it connects your ability to accept others and new experiences. It is the source of your feelings, and when it is **in balance**, it brings grace, flexibility, fulfilment, and creativity.

Signs & Symptoms of Imbalanced Sacral Chakra:

- Overeating
- Emotional Oversensitivity
- Guilt
- Apathy
- Creativity Blocks
- Detachment
- Codependency
- Guilt

Visualize a beam of orange light glowing below your belly button and affirm the following:

- I am radiant, beautiful, and strong
- I am in touch with my feelings

- I am alive, connected, and aware
- I acknowledge my authenticity and uniqueness; there is only one of me
- I embrace life with joy and happiness and follow my passions
- I am a beautiful person and full of creative potential

Chakra 3: Solar Plexus

The solar plexus is located above the belly button, below the heart, and its color is yellow. It is the center of the energy associated with ego and is the source of self-belief, self-worth, and personal power. Signs of being **in balance** and open are a healthy self-esteem, strong will power, happiness, faith in the future, self-belief, ambition, drive, healthy ego, self confidence.

Signs & Symptoms of Imbalanced Solar Plexus Chakra

- Life becomes a series of disappointments and frustrations
- Self-victimization
- Pessimism
- Low Expectations & Life Aspirations
- Lack of Self-Worth
- Low Self-Esteem
- Passiveness

Visualize a bright yellow light glowing above your belly button below your heart and affirm the following:

- I am confident in all that I do
- I choose health, healing and happiness
- I stand up for myself
- I act with courage and strength
- I am connected to the abundant flow of the universe and easily manifest my dreams
- I have all the ingredients and resources to manifest my dreams and desires

Chakra 4: Heart

The heart chakra is green, and it connects us to our emotional health, and brings love, forgiveness and gratitude from within. When **in balance,** you will feel loving, kind, empathetic, compassionate to yourself and others, as well as be forgiving, happy for others success, joyful, abundant, emotionally balanced, trusting, and able to give and receive love.

Signs & Symptoms of Imbalanced Heart Chakra:

- Demanding Personality
- Critical of self & others
- Judgmental
- Jealous
- Insecure
- Lonely
- Manipulative
- Cold-Hearted
- Malicious
- Negative

Visualize green from your heart and affirm the following:

- I live in balance, in a state of gracefulness and gratitude
- I am grateful for all the challenges that helped me transform and grow into a better version of myself
- I am loved
- I am fully open to giving love
- I am fully open to receiving love
- I forgive myself
- I forgive others

Chakra 5: Throat

The beaming blue throat chakra is located at the throat and is affected by your thoughts and feelings related to speaking the truth, and talking to yourself, loved ones, family, friends, customers, and coworkers with kindness and compassion, communicating with honesty, and asking for your needs to be met. It really impacts your ability to speak to yourself and others. When **in balance**, we express ourselves fully without caring what others think (in a nice way, of course), and are honest to ourselves and others.

Signs & Symptoms of Imbalanced Throat Chakra

- Fear
- Worry about expressing and communicating the truth
- Issues with self-expression and inner confidence

A great way to honor your throat chakra is to do a daily mind dump on paper to help empty your worries and fears.

Focus on your throat, visualize blue, and affirm the following:

- I am aligned with my highest truth
- I communicate the truth with love and honor
- I express myself fully, showing my true colors
- I am connected to my true path and purpose
- All of the answers I need are inside of me
- I easily hear the voice of my soul

Chakra 6: Third Eye

Your third eye is located between your eyebrow and forehead and is associated with the colour indigo. It connects you to your cosmic insight and intuition. When it's **in balance**, you will feel a deep spiritual connection, be open, focused on dreams and desires, follow your gut instincts, gain ability to think, mental clarity, peaceful dreams, forgiveness of others, and you will be spiritually awake.

Signs & Symptoms of Imbalanced Third Eye Chakra

- Mood swings
- Uncertainty about life path

- Clouded vision of future
- Lack of motivation
- No hope for the future or present

Visualize the color indigo beaming from your third eye point and affirm the following:

- I expand my awareness through my inner self
- I am insightful and intuitive
- I always follow and honor my intuition
- My thoughts are calm and peaceful
- I have a healthy mind
- I have a creative imagination
- I pay attention to signs and messages from my soul

Chakra 7: Crown

The crown chakra is the 7th chakra, located at the top of the head. It is purple, and when it's in balance, it's the source of enlightenment, spiritual connection, inspiration, positivity, happiness, devotion, trust in your higher self, living fully in the present, and living in a conscious state of mind.

Signs & Symptoms of Imbalanced Crown Chakra

- Closed mindedness
- Disconnected from real self
- Frustration
- Spiritually Unaware
- Rigid
- Depression
- Inability to see the bigger picture
- Negative Mental Chatter

Visualize purple at the crown of your head and affirm the following:

- I am worthy of love from divine energy

- I am a being of love and light
- I go beyond my limiting beliefs
- I seek experiences that nourish my spirit
- I am connected to my purpose
- I trust that I am loved completely and unconditionally

Body Positivity

As you can see, I use the P-Word (positive) a lot throughout this book, but it really is paramount to vitality, energy and true radiance from within. I want to touch on the topic of body positivity, something that is part of a recent movement due to social media domination.

Side note: I use social media and think it is an incredible platform to connect with like-minded people and spread your message; however, with all the intense filters, edits, and "perfect" lifestyle pics around, it can be extremely disheartening for those who are not feeling so great about themselves. Now that I have a daughter myself, I am more aware of the importance of body positivity, especially considering a whopping 70 percent of younger girls feel insecure about themselves, which mostly comes from social media and the obsession of pop culture and celebrities.

Be in love with who you are, and I mean every single part of you—you are a beautiful being and are unique in your own right. Begin to pay attention and focus on the highs of yourself rather than the lows. Are you curvy and have a bigger bust? Well, that's amazing! Be proud of that. Are you smaller built and petite? Love that and embrace it too!

Whatever shape or size you are, begin to love that, and STOP, stop, **stop** comparing yourself to anyone else. As you implement beauty food feasting into your lifestyle, you will feel light, happy, and healthy from within, and when you carve out time for regular movement, you will begin, to sculpt, strengthen and tone your body, which will boost inner confidence naturally. So instead of scrolling through super models' images, or over filtered accounts you follow, focus on your health. Comparing yourself to others is not good for your inner beauty and health. When you nourish your mind, body, and spirit from the inside out, you will naturally feel positive about yourself. From this day forward FU** those nasty negative harmful thoughts about yourself, and OWN who you are, love every bit, and that will shine from within. Start to visualize how you want to feel and look like, and will become reality before you know it.

Ashfab Social Media Tip: unfollow every account, that makes you feel bad about yourself and makes you want to be someone else other than the beautiful you.

> **"Have a beautiful, healthy, positive vision filled with a grateful heart, and that is what you will feel and experience."**
>
> **—Ashley Siedentopf**

Remember, life is precious and the people in your life are what will make it a happier, and healthier internally. Stay positive, be grateful, use uplifting affirmations, meditate daily, practice yoga, get your beauty sleep surround yourself with people that bring out the most fab version of you, and be kind, compassionate, and loving to yourself. More importantly, creating a life you love comes from total commitment to personal growth and personal development, and it takes daily time and effort.

Overview for Feeling Fab

- **Think, act, and switch to a positive mindset.**
- **Adopt an attitude of gratitude, learn to appreciate even the smallest things, and jot them down daily**
- **Surround yourself with uplifting, sincere, kind, fun-loving, people**
- **Affirm awesome thoughts about yourself**
- **Meditate every day**
- **Get your beauty sleep at least 8–9 hours a night (this does not apply to new mums with small babies)**
- **Use organic essential oils**
- **Start yoga or continue to deepen your practice**
- **Stay motivated**
- **Follow your joy**

- Love thyself
- Spread healthy vibes
- Keep your chakras open, aligned and activated, to feel balanced, positive and energised from within.
- Adjust your mindset
- Focus on body positivity

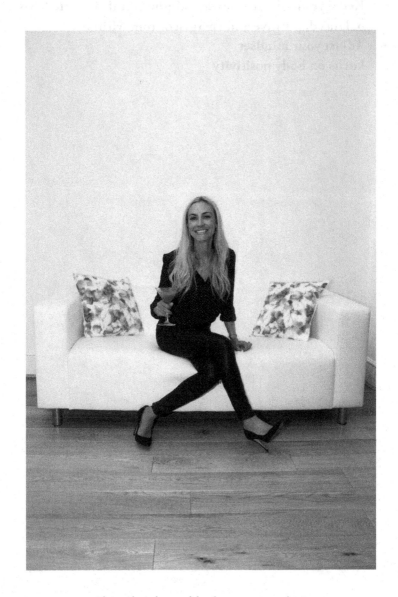

Shine bright and be happy everyday!

PART 3

Live Fab

Living fabulously requires a mindset that is free from negative thoughts, enthusiastic about life, and excited about today. The key is focusing on the present, having a positive attitude, and feeling confident, bold, and energetic.

Modern-day living can be stressful. Smartphones can be soul-sucking, and social media can make you forget to live in the moment. Instead of appreciating the beauty around you, you forget to live fully in this moment. Taking an optimistic approach in life will help you live a fabulous life beyond your wildest dreams.

We only have one life. It is a privilege itself to get to wake up each morning with a new chance to be here and live. All it takes is to learn to live in the present and make peace with your life by bringing more awareness to your wellbeing and simply being here now.

Top Tips for Living Life in the Fab Lane

Follow your dreams

As children, we have no worries. We constantly dream, create, play, and use our imaginations. With not a worry in the sky, our minds are free from any fears, negative blocks, or nasty thoughts. We only have one life; today is the present, tomorrow is the future, and yesterday becomes the past. We should go through life as we did when we were children by living for today and doing something that makes us feel fulfilled, purposeful, and motivated.

Following your dreams is simpler than it sounds. Think about your passions. What makes your heart sing and your eyes light up? What are you interested in? What kind of books and magazines do you like to read? What are some of your skills? How would you describe yourself in five words? Write down answers to these questions, and you will start to see a pattern.

Know this: your passion and your talent can become your dream job eventually if you set your mind to it. It won't happen overnight, but it will happen. Pay attention to your thoughts and the messages you receive. Focus and take action. Stay motivated by taking short courses to help you explore different options, and observe the role models around you. These steps will get you closer to your dreams.

Maybe you want to open a bakery or wellness studio, write a novel, launch a blog related to your interests, or go back to school to study something that interests you. Follow your dreams, pursue your passions, expand your horizons, and gain experience, because if you refuse to give up on your dreams and continue to have faith and belief in them, you will do what you love, and love what you do in time. **Life is for living, so live it fabulously.**

> **"You don't have forever to wait for people and dreams to come true. You must move towards them. You can't spend your life reacting to the world and waiting for it to magically heal all your wounds and give you everything you want. You must. You must make choices to reflect that your time and your life matter. Eat great food. Exercise. Love the vessel you were given. Pursue your passions and your gifts. Open your heart at every moment. And, most importantly, don't leave anything unloved, including yourself."**
>
> **—Mark Groves**

Face your fears

Life can sometimes feel a little stale. Maybe you lost your mojo or feel less than enthused about the current state you are in, whether it's a relationship that has lost its spark, a career that no longer fulfills you, or just general life that has become boring and unexciting. It is important to set aside some time alone; figure out what is no longer supporting growth, inner peace, happiness, or joy.

Check in with yourself to see what areas of life need improvement and what it is you need to do to change it. Maybe it's building the courage to end that not-so-healthy relationship or quitting your job to set up the cupcake shop you always dreamed of. Maybe moving to a new country could be the key to reinventing yourself by helping you find your purpose and face your fears.

The goal is to get closer to the most fab version of yourself, and to have faith everything will work out. Ask yourself, "What would I want to do if I don't have to worry about the 'what-ifs,' financial constraints, or just general fear and doubt that it won't work out?"

For just a moment, try to forget all the what-ifs and worries. Take money and worst-case scenarios out of the picture. Open your heart and imagine the highest, grandest visions of yourself. Feeling those positive emotions will truly get you closer to your dream. When there is a will, there is a way, so for the first time, just think of what YOU want to do — not how it's going happen or who is going to judge you or whether or not it's a good idea.

The more you remove your fears of failure, self-limitations, and doubt from your vocabulary, and instead focus on the on the prize, have faith in the future, and embrace positive emotions about the outcome, the sooner it will become a reality. You have to be your own cheerleader — have complete hope, belief, and faith in yourself and future.

Let go of any past struggles or setbacks that may have heightened any fearful thoughts. Be patient with the present, as things don't happen overnight, and be excited about your future. Fear, doubt, and disbelief are only going to sabotage our pathway to success. And when I speak of success, I don't just mean, a big bank account, a huge house, or a nice car; I mean a sense of fulfilment in all areas of your life.

If it helps, write it on post it notes or get a colorful felt pen and write inspiring quotes on your mirror. Furthermore, having confidence is key in your next move. Confident people are authentic, not afraid to express themselves, and live by their own rules.

Don't compare yourself to others. Focus on your qualities and try to improve your weaknesses. Nobody is perfect! Whether you want to get a promotion, lose those extra 5 pounds, start your own business, or leave an outdated relationship, believe in yourself because you can do anything you put your mind to. Replace negative talk with positive affirmations.

Whenever you catch yourself thinking negative thoughts, reverse it to say something positive instead:

- Instead of "I feel unattractive," say, "I am beautiful."
- Instead of "I don't have the skills," say, "I believe I can do anything I put my mind to."

It may not feel believable at first, but repeat these positive mantras regularly, and you'll begin to see yourself in the new light.

When I wake up in the morning, I jot down a positive thought, intention, or mantra in my big journal. Next, I write out a realistic to-do list, followed by three things I am grateful for. I started doing this September 2012 and it has had a profound effect on my life. It not only gives me a sense of clarity and contentment, but it also boosts my productivity and positive outlook for the day.

By dedicating your time and energy into self-belief, self-love, and self-care, you will feel happier, more joyful, uplifted, peaceful, positive, and loving. You need to flex that muscle every single day. The more you work on removing fear from your life, the more your life will flourish. Think what you want, speak about it, act on it, and feel it by having faith everything will work out.

Don't even let fear be an option. Next time you are faced with something that could cause jitters or self-doubt, just be brave and know it's ok to screw up and grow from it. Fear is just created by our imagination, so ditch the feeling from your inner vocabulary.

"Every great dream begins with a dreamer. Always remember, you have within you the strength, the patience, and the passion to reach for the stars to change the world."

—Harriet Tubman

Surround yourself with art

Art comes in all forms, from painting and photography to yoga, travel, theatre, opera, dance, books, writing, film, fashion, and food. **"Art is a diverse range of human activities in creating visual, auditory or performing artefacts — artworks, expressing the author's imaginative or technical skill, intended to be appreciated for their beauty or**

emotional power." Here are some ways to get a little more oomph in your life with art:

- Read at least 10 books a year on self-improvement, development, success, happiness, or life inspiration. Reading gives you more brain power and it strengthens your skills. It can even unleash hidden thoughts or talents!
- Check out exhibitions focused on art and fashion to help you appreciate beauty
- Travel to at least one new place a year. Take in the scenery, culture, food, and fun. Living like a local is way more interesting than doing typical tourist activities
- Watch foreign films. Or watch a comedy to help you switch off and be entertained
- Write a letter to an old friend, a poem to a loved one, or article on something that you are passionate about. Writing helps with creativity and self-expression, which has always been essential to our humanity, or get out your crayons and enjoy an afternoon of colouring
- If you are new to yoga, book a beginner class! Yoga is an amazing form of exercise that clears your head and helps you be more mindful. Some people even say they feel more enlightened, which helps them move into a direction of their dreams

Pursue whatever type of art interests you, whether it's watching, reading, writing, seeing, doing, exploring, taking photographs, or looking at pictures. Art helps build self-esteem, increases motivation, and improves focus and communication. It can even strengthen your relationship with the environment.

> **"You are the books you read, the films you watch, the music you listen to, the people you meet, the dreams you have, and the conversation you engage in. You are what you take from these. You are the sound of the ocean, the breath of fresh air, the brightest light, and the darkest corner. You are a collection of every experience you have had in your life. You are every**

single second of every single day. So, drown yourself in a sea of knowledge and existence. Let the words run through your veins and let the colors fill your mind until there is nothing left to do but explode. There are no wrong answers. Inspiration is everywhere. Sit back, relax, and take it all in. Now go out and create something."

Unknown

Discover your passions

Passion is what lights us up, makes us feel good, and keeps our lives enriched. To put it simply, I am passionate about life, organic healthy living, cooking, spirituality, skincare, wine, wellness, fashion, photography, real estate, interior design, and travel. I love laughing, living in the moment, being spontaneous, having fun, being excited about being excited, and living every day fully. I am an advocate for organic healthy living. It feeds my mind, body, and soul. It gives me energy, keeps me well, and has transformed my health significantly, making me want to inspire others to take a holistic approach to health.

I took my first long flight at six weeks old to the UK from Canada and have not stopped since. I always love the thrill of arriving at a new destination. I enjoy living like the locals and learning about where they hang out, eat, drink, dance, etc. I love exploring new cultures and worldly flavors, and because I grew up in Canada and have lived in Europe for 15 years, I now constantly crave sun, sand, and sea. I love tropical trips but also enjoy a weekend city break to NYC or Paris now and then.

I try to align my desires and values with my passions, which keeps me feeling upbeat about what I do and why I am doing it. To give you a glimpse of what you are passionate about, think of your interests, hobbies, and whatever you feel enthusiastic about. For example, what types of magazines or books are you drawn to? What kind of websites do you find yourself browsing during your down time?

Now take a moment, close your eyes, and take note of the first three things that pop into your head. Write them down on a piece of paper and put it somewhere that is visible. Whatever you are doing in your life, find time to follow or pursue your passions. Be conscious and present, and pay attention to thoughts and messages.

We have one life, and one life only. It is entirely up to us to make the most of it, so make time for your passions. You never know what could happen in the future. This doesn't mean you have to turn your passion into a full-time job, but spending time doing things that you are passionate about will feed your soul and make you feel good. Things that we imagine and daydream about can be insightful and show us what could become reality. Pay attention to intuition, whispers of the soul, and messages. Make time for things that light you up and give you a deep sense of joy and happiness.

Focus on what you have

If you are constantly focusing on things you do not have or thinking about how you are not where you currently want to be, it will suck the joy out of your life and take away all the goodness and beauty that already surrounds you. It will prevent you from being able to appreciate all the things that you do have.

What you focus on expands and grows, both negative and positive, so if you are constantly complaining about not having enough, your job, or your weight — the list could go on — you will keep experiencing negative karma. Instead, train your brain to focus on what you want and to appreciate what you have. Affirm it, and soon, abundance will surround you!

For example, imagine that someone gave you one macaroon, not three. If you focus on how you wanted three but only got one, you won't be able to enjoy the macaroon that you did receive. This way of thinking will never allow you to enjoy the macaroon you have. So, it is really important to appreciate the things which you have rather than simply yearning for what you don't have.

Whatever you give thanks for in your life, you will get more of it. Having a "lack of" mentality and being ungrateful for the simple things in life is only going to hinder your path of love, joy, and freedom, so start to acknowledge how lucky you are and give thanks to all that you have. This will have a huge positive effect on your life.

Just like anyone else, yes, I would love more shoes, bags, and jewels, but I am happy with what I do have. Eventually, I'm sure, my wardrobe will grow, and so will my smile, since I am grateful for the simple things in life, like a warm home, good health, a supportive family, my amazing husband, wellness treatments, good food, travel, fun experiences, and great friends.

Simply continue to count your blessings and focus on what you do have rather than what you do not have. Give thanks for all that you have in your life every single day and begin to look around for all the goodness that surrounds you, because what you focus on grows. Focus on the good, think about what you want, affirm it often, and you will get more of that!

> **"If you can't stop thinking about it, don't stop working for it."**
>
> **Unknown**

Beautify your brain

My beauty food feasting approach has a positive impact on your brain health, which leads to better mood and memory in the long run. However, feeling more focused, switched on, savvy, motivated, and inspired requires you to keep using your brain and learning from experts in spirituality, positivity, motivation, success, and leadership.

I suggest reading something inspirational and educational for at least 20 minutes every night before bed. By flexing these brain muscles over time, you wake up feeling more motivated, inspired, and excited for the day, as you have gone to sleep with something uplifting that stays in the subconscious part of your brain. Save the juicy Jackie Collins or thriller books for holidays or downtime on weekends. During the week, make an effort to read materials that teach you about life, success, spirituality, personal growth, and the like. By doing this, you will increase your sense of well-being and day-to-day living.

If reading doesn't fit into your schedule, try audiobooks while walking or driving in the car. Another way to boost your brain power and nourish your subconscious health-positive emotions is by listening to inspiring podcasts. This can easily be done while you're driving to work, on the tube, doing your makeup, or cooking. You can explore whatever you want in as little as 10 minutes a day and try to explore books on spirituality, success, psychology, health, leadership, happiness, and mindfulness. It will only boost your overall sense of health and wellbeing.

It doesn't matter how old you are — never stop learning. Commit to carving out time to boost your brain power. Some of my greatest teachers that have been paramount to my inner work journey are Oprah Winfrey, Deepak Chopra, Louise Hay, Marriam Williamson, Wayne Dyer, and Fiona Harold. If you're not sure where to start, try reading materials written by some of these amazing teachers.

Other ways to nourish and optimize your brain to improve focus, clarity, and concentration is by taking ginkgo biloba, ginseng, gaba, 5 HTP, CBD oil, and of course, high quality fish oils.

"Stay interested to be interesting."

—Dr. Murad

Always wear your invisible crown.

Feeling confident is the first step to feeling fabulous. If you're not feeling your most confident, don't worry. None of us are born confident. Some people are more confident than others, which could possibly stem from early childhood; however, it is never too late to feel and become the confident woman (or person) you can be. The key to confidence is believing, affirming, and knowing you are fabulous, amazing, and beautiful every single day, having faith in all areas of your life, and believing in yourself wholeheartedly.

Affirming awesome thoughts about yourself, reminding yourself how beautiful you are, and being confident requires time and effort from yourself. No one is a better confidence coach than yourself, so you must be your own cheerleader, and remember all the unique qualities and strengths you have! When doubt and low self-esteem creep in, simply zap the thought with three positive thoughts, and tell yourself out loud, how fabulous, amazing, and beautiful you are. Always wear invisible crown, stand tall, walk with pride, speak with confidence, and remember: in the world, there is only one of you!

You ultimately become what you believe and think. Whether they're big or small, those thoughts become your reality, so you might as well have the highest, grandest visions and opinions of yourself. So, go on, and think the most loving, nourishing thoughts about yourself that will radiate and glow from within.

Confident people are authentic. They're not afraid to express themselves and live by their own rules; not to mention, they have the ability to trust and believe they can do anything. Don't compare yourself to others; focus on your qualities and try to improve on your weaknesses. Nobody is perfect. We are all human and carry flaws, but really, it just comes down to trying to be the best we can be today. My best friend Amanda, one of my most confident friends, once told me if she ever has a moment of doubt about herself, she remembers the following quote:

"Only when we are no longer afraid do we begin to live."

—Dorothy Thompson

Learn how to say no

I was the queen of saying yes to everything not so long ago. In the past, I would always end up saying yes to all social events and engagements or entertaining every visitor that would come through London, only to feel completely frazzled and burned out. Making self-care a priority also made me shift my mindset to only saying yes to things I truly wanted to do, that made me happy, and gave me a sense of joy.

It has taken me time to learn how to say no to things that I deep down didn't want to do, or felt more like a chore. So now if something feels like, "Ughhhh, do I *have* to?" it is much easier for me to just say no. Time is just so precious, and as we get older, life becomes busier, so commit your time to things you really want to do, things that bring good energy and happiness to your life. Bottom line: put you and your priorities first. Your dearest friends and family will understand and still love you. :-)

Declutter your life

I am sure you all have done some kind of decluttering, or at least thrown out a T-shirt or two from high school that you haven't worn in over a decade (at least it's a start!). But I am talking about a decluttering process from head to toe, from the bedroom to your bathroom, or from your books to your beauty products.

One of the best ways to maximize your productivity is to do a big clearing out of your home. Your surroundings are a reflection of you, so think: a cluttered house equals a cluttered mind, and an organized house equals an organized mind.

Envision how you would like the end result to look. Think of why you want to clean and what it will look like. Find ways to get rid of things you don't need anymore. Donate your items to local charity shops, friends, or eBay.

Next, **create a list.** Step by step, check it off as you complete each section. Doing this will help motivate you to complete the project.

Give yourself a realistic timeline. Take small breaks so you don't get overwhelmed or discouraged, and **start somewhere small** that will still make a big difference, like the bathroom. Make a list from old outdated beauty products, books, clothes, shoes, electronics, books to kitchen stuff, clothes, shoes, undies, DVDs, home office supplies, etc. Simply go through these items, giving 100 percent of your focus to each particular area or category.

I love to declutter seasonally. It makes room for new purchases and prevents the mind going into chaotic overload.

> **"Being out of balance can have significant effects on all aspects of your life. Create harmony in your life and establish a healthy rhythm that is sustainable and feels good to you."**
>
> **—Institute of Integrative Nutrition**

Believe in yourself

Whatever it is you want to achieve and accomplish in your life, whether it's carving a new career path, moving to a new country, or having a dream body, they all have something in common: they are require self-belief, which translates to constantly reminding yourself you can do it, and *knowing* you can do it.

Believing in yourself will put your mind into a super-focused visionary thinking mode, so when you combine **self-belief** plus **daily action** plus **focus** plus **not losing sight of your vision**, I guarantee you will be where you want to be in time.

Beliefs we hold about ourselves can either hinder or help our success. Act as if, whatever it is you want to achieve *will* come true. Don't use the old saying, "I'll believe it when I see it." Instead, it is better to truly think and feel, "I see it and believe it." If you reached your goals today, how would you feel? How would you dress? Act? Think? Speak? Act now as if you have already achieved this goal.

We all have something we want in life that may feel out of reach at this time; however, by adopting the right mindset and believing in yourself whole-heartedly, you are saying, "screw you" to self-doubt. Whatever your goal is, you should feel, act, and believe you are a success today, and whatever you do, never lose sight of this vision.

> **"What you are drawn to — that is your soul speaking to you."**
>
> **— Unknown**

> **"Your smile is your logo, your personality is your business card, and how you leave others after an experience with you becomes your trademark, so don't be afraid to be unique."**
>
> **Unknown**

Practice self-care

Self-care is truly the best healthcare. Putting yourself and health first will have a huge impact on your relationships, work, and family members. If you are constantly putting other people and other events before yourself, you will start feeling overwhelmed, anxious, stressed, and out of balance. Set aside time for yourself for the things you love, like yoga, reading, a reiki, acupuncture, journaling, visualization, aromatherapy, or an afternoon at the spa. The more you nourish yourself with things you love, the more you can give love to your surroundings.

Meditation, a massage, yoga, and brisk walks in nature are f.a.b ways to give that time to yourself to switch off and clear out mental clutter. It's important to prioritize yourself and protect your energy, so don't feel guilty about cancelling a commitment, taking a day off, doing nothing, or even turning your phone off and switching off from social media. Make self-care priority number one so that you can feel well and thrive in all areas of your life.

Self-care is not just a luxury; it is an absolute necessity and should be a top priority in your wellness regime. Whether you're solo or surrounded by a big family, self-care must come first. It is not selfish; it is selfless. When you feel healthy, you can give your best to all other areas of life including work, home, relationships, fitness, spirituality, etc.

There are infinite ways you can make time for self-care. This includes filling your body with wholesome foods to boost both your health and inner beauty on a daily basis. Make a promise to yourself to make self-care a sacred part of your life. By putting yourself first, you will experience tremendous emotional, physical, and mental health benefits.

In my experience, when I take care of myself, I feel more balanced, and I'm less prone to cold, flu, and infections. I am less stressed and, ultimately, I feel more vibrant, energetic, and happier. Many people sacrifice their self-care in the modern-day world due to the stresses of daily life — having a hectic schedule, over working, and essentially taking on too much — which can leave us feeling sick, tired, stressed, and uncared for. Self-care is simply the best healthcare you can do. It is vital to your health, beauty, and wellbeing. If we pile too much on our plate and always put loved ones first, eventually, we just end up feeling burned out, stressed, resentful, and plain old imbalanced.

By affirming every day how amazing you are, you naturally give yourself an inner boost of confidence and clarity. Self-love and self-belief are both forms of self-care. By making the relationship with yourself your number one priority, learning to love and embrace everything about you, and believing in yourself and your ability to achieve whatever it is you want to do in this world, you will encourage your mindset to spend more time in self-care, self-love and self-belief mode.

All of these tips in this book are, in fact, forms of self-care, because ultimately you need to nourish to flourish from the inside out. That means truly taking care of yourself with nutrition, movement, mindset, and things that bring you joy so that your self-care battery is always fully charged. Begin to pay attention to when it is low, and carve out some extra time for yourself to reset your system, and bring inner peace and balance.

From this day forward, try to remind yourself of the importance of self-care. Slow down and prioritize yourself. Be mindful of your thoughts, actions, and deeds. Rest when you need to, and get the support and comfort you need. Simply just be here, now.

Put yourself first by creating a healthy relationship with yourself, and your health and happiness will thrive in all areas of your life. It's OK to cancel plans. It is okay to have an evening of pajamas, pizza, and at-home pampering, if you need it. Listen to your body. Rest, and slow down when you need to, and by no means feel guilty about it. Make a promise to yourself to make self-care a sacred part of your life to optimize your health, wellbeing, and beauty from the inside out.

When it comes down to it, most of these tips are types of self-care, since they help you care for yourself on all levels, from the inside out. When you make self-care the most important thing in your life, you will truly take back your power and potential.

Self-Care Ideas

- Book a massage
- Put on a face mask

- Soak in the tub and light a scented candle
- Get a mani-pedi
- Tuck yourself into bed with a good book and a cup of herbal tea
- Go for a walk in nature
- Buy yourself flowers
- Try restorative-style yoga
- Cook a nourishing meal
- Do a social media detox for a day
- Meditate
- Go to bed early
- Watch the sunset
- Journal out any dream, desires, and worries
- Say no to a social commitment when you feel like staying home
- Declutter your clothes and give them to charity
- Listen to a motivational podcast
- Create a morning and nighttime routine
- Do some gardening
- Get a blowout to give you an instant beauty boost

Be more mindful

Mindfulness has made a big wave around the world over the last few years. More and more people are making it an important part of their health and wellness regime. Being mindful requires you to be in tune with your breath, thoughts, feelings, and surroundings.

When you begin to practice mindfulness, your main focus should be on being here, now. Live in the present, pay attention to what is currently happening, and simply be aware of the beauty that surrounds you. The more you become mindful of your thoughts, feelings, breaths, and behaviour he lighter your mind, body, soul, and spirit will feel. You will feel more connected and aligned to your true self.

It is important to not be harsh or judgmental toward your own thoughts. Mindfulness does require dedication and determination; however, with practice, you will begin to make more of an effort to be mindful of your thoughts, breaths, and feelings. You start to manage mental, emotional, and spiritual health with mindfulness, helping you feel more joyful, happier, uplifted, enthusiastic, and peaceful from within. When you begin to change your thoughts from the inside and become more conscious and self-aware, you will see a profound effect on the outer aspects of your life.

Set aside time for mediation. Meditating first-thing in the morning is a great way to begin your day, however 20 minutes midday or before bed is as effective. Wake up, find a quiet spot, and focus on breathing slowly and deeply. Other forms of stillness can be while you drink your tea or coffee or enjoy a meal. Savor the moment, sip slowly, chew thoroughly, and take breaks in between bites, blessing each moment. Go outside every day for a brisk walk and look for all the beauty and any nature that surrounds you.

Count your blessings in the morning and before you sleep, appreciating what you have — expressing gratitude daily will bring you joy and a sense of fulfilment instantly. There are so many reasons to be grateful. Start by appreciating the small things, and simply just be. Become more aware of your thoughts, feelings, and the current moment. Go at a pace that suits you in life, and practice yoga. Yoga combines breathing, moving, and meditating, so you'll feel amazing when you do it. Focus on breath work, get your heart rate up, stretch out your body, and release tension held around your hips or in your shoulders. Find a style that suits you, and try it a few times a week. Yoga is a wonderful workout for your mind, body, soul, and spirit.

Mindfulness requires discipline, dedication, and devotion to your inside health. Start by doing daily body scans. Think about how you're feeling, whether it's light or heavy, happy or sad, anxious or calm. Shift your thoughts to happier ones by breathing slowly and bringing awareness to your mind, body, and spirit. Improve your thoughts and become healthier mentally and physically. One brilliant app that I recently discovered is INSIGHT timer. Check it out if you want to start to introduce more mindfulness into your life — you won't regret it.

Self-love + positive vibes – negativity + a grateful heart = the holy grail of happiness

Stay mentally motivated

Staying motivated during your new path to vibrant health, natural beauty, and inner well- being requires discipline, dedication, and doing something every day to bring you closer to your goals. Motivation is the force that guides our behaviors to get results.

Believing and visualizing how you want to look and feel means you're already half-way there, so set a goal to visualize it down to the last detail! See it, feel it, eat it, and breathe it. When you focus on the outcome, you will automatically feel more excited and energized to do whatever it is you need to do.

While you're on this path to fabulosity, implement the 3 Ps: stay positive, patient, and persistent. Adopt an upbeat, grateful, positive attitude, and do not compare yourself to others. Being motivated takes daily action, having a deep level of focus, and making small steps toward your goal. This is vital to your success.

Glow like a goddess

Now that you understand the power of plants, positivity, staying present, and powerful beliefs about yourself, it is time to start thinking like a goddess! Remind yourself how beautiful and unique you are; focus on your strengths, work on your weaknesses, and learn to honor and treat your body as a temple.

Free your mind from negative thoughts, spend time alone, and listen to your inner voice. Pay attention to signs and messages you hear and see. This could be your calling! Be strong in your mind, be brave, stand tall, and walk, talk, and think beautifully with love, grace, and gratitude.

Learn more about your moon sign and star sign. Your star sign is the more masculine Yang, and your moon sign is the more feminine Yin. It is important to understand them both, so you feel fully balanced and beautiful.

My star sign is Aries and my moon sign is Virgo, so try I to focus on the good qualities that come with both. The downside of Aries is that we can be slightly impulsive and aggressive, while Virgos can be overly critical and analytical. If I ever experience these not-so-great qualities that are not goddess-worthy, I focus on the good, uplifting energy of the Aries, a pioneer, trailblazing warrior at heart, and on the good qualities of Virgo, which are precision, femininity, and modesty. This helps me put things in order and center myself. I become aware of my thoughts and feelings, and I feel back to "Ashley" in no time.

It is really important to connect with your spiritual side to truly feel like a glowing goddess. Learning about and understanding your star and moon signs also helps you get a better understanding of yourself, bringing out the best in you.

Unleash your creativity, and go for walks in nature. Express your true emotions in a graceful way. Meditate daily, write in your journal, and pay attention to signs and messages. Make friends and bond with fellow fabulous females. All of these steps will help you feel and think like a goddess. Putting yourself first is not selfish — **it's selfless** because it allows you to give 100 percent of your effort to your loved ones.

Dare to dream and unleash the goddess within. When you start to love yourself wholeheartedly, be more authentic, love your flaws, embrace your imperfections and vulnerabilities, and are comfortable in your own skin, your inner goddess will really shine.

"Real women fix each other's crowns."

Unknown

Stay present

Simply be here, now, for this moment. Try not to fret about the future or dwell on the past; slow down and enjoy the present. Be patient with the present and grateful for the journey you are on. Yesterday is gone and the future is not here yet! By living in the NOW, you will begin to shift that negative attitude to a positive one, because living in the NOW makes you focus your thoughts on the importance of the present.

Of course, we all have those moments, perhaps before you go to bed, or on your way to work where you think "what if" or "why did I do that?" Dwelling on these things will not benefit you in any way and will instead block the flow of fab abundance. It's time to learn to get in the driver's seat and be in control of your own thoughts and mind.

Living in the future makes you feel anxious, while living in the past makes you feel depressed; however, living in the present makes you feel at peace, so be here now. Live in the moment, and simply just take a few deep breaths. Set aside some time for some serious self-care if you're feeling a little low or slightly anxious. When you begin to notice the beauty in everything, slow down, take time out, and implement meditation into your health regime, your mind will naturally become more present.

When you have negative thoughts about the past or the future, it can prevent you from living in the moment. Of course, it can be healthy to reminisce and think of great memories of your past, and dream and get excited about new endeavors in the future, but make sure they are healthy thoughts, and train your brain to be here now, today, fully present and positive. The more self-aware you become, the more you will be able to control those not-so-fabifying thoughts and feelings.

Fall in love with your life

Become a life lover. By this, I mean value and cherish each day, as if it is your last. This motto has been part of my life since my teens, from spending a lot of time sick in the hospital, to surviving a near fatal experience when I was 24. The times I spent in the hospital definitely had an impact on me mentally and inspired me to live life fully and become a life-lover.

Death is truly our greatest teacher, and at any moment, our life could be taken away. Let's not wait for those times to come. Do not take the time you have left for granted. Ideally, we hopefully live a long, healthy, fruitful life. Don't stop having fun while you are here. I am all for taking your work seriously, but yourself and your life? Not so much.

Think, feel, and act as if we might experience our last moments and inhale our last breaths of air on earth at any time. Soak up different types of experiences. Stay on the path of beauty, love, joy, peace, and appreciation. Forgive others, let go of grudges, and be kind to everyone. Be nice, stop judging others and yourself. It's all just a waste of negative energy, mental clutter, and spiritual debris.

Connect with mother nature, music, and close friends often. Just waking up and shifting your mindset to a "life-lover" will have a domino effect on your everyday experience. When you love life, life will love you right back.

Although I was diagnosed with Crohn's disease 24 years ago, hospitalized many times in the past, and had a horrific near-death experience in Athens, living with an illness still today and experiencing those difficult times made me a better, kinder, more compassionate person, I'm still far from perfect, but I try to be the best version of me and to others.

It's like when I was hit with an illness at a young age. This terrifying, nearly fatal experience really woke me up. I truly believe it brought out my free spirit nature, find the best in people, and appreciate the gift of life itself. That said, by no means do you have to wait for an illness like this to start loving your life!

"Joie de vivré"

When I lived and worked in St. Tropez for over four months 12 years ago, I picked up a phrase that forever stuck with me, and that was "joie de vivré" which translates to "exuberant excitement of life" or "a feeling of great happiness and enjoyment of life."

Life is so precious, and time goes by so quickly, especially as we get older. It is so important to slow down, look around you, be excited about life, and find little things to celebrate often.

If you are reading this and not feeling so excited, make a list of things that you love doing to spark that excitement, even if it is just calling some girlfriends up and arranging a nice dinner to get together, or making plans with a friend to go to the farmers market on Saturday followed by brunch. Or even better, book a much-needed holiday.

Most people only like to celebrate if they have gotten a big promotion, a raise, or a ring on their finger. These big life moments are of course reason to celebrate; however, I mean to celebrate often. When I walk my dog in the morning to get coffee, I am celebrating that moment, being healthy and able to walk, and being able to pay for premium coffee. Celebrating isn't just about popping champagne for a special occasion; it's celebrating life through food, friends, experiences, and deep gratitude, remembering that the gift of life itself is a privilege and a special occasion.

Your presence is your power

No one can ever replace the power of your presence but yourself. When you walk into a room or are introduced to others for the first time, within 10 seconds, your presence either makes an impact or it doesn't. I'm not saying you have to be a loud, proud, bold, extroverted look-at-me kind of person walking around with a microphone; what I'm saying is that a warm, sincere, approachable, real presence sends out way more positive vibes, than a cold, standoffish, not-so-happy presence. As you are growing into the greatest version of yourself from the inside out, you will naturally become more aware of your thoughts, patterns, vibes, and of course, presence.

So, embrace your personality and fully become you. Let your true traits shine through, and don't dwell on perfection — none of us are perfect. We are all human and have flaws. However, we all have pretty amazing parts about us too. Know what your strengths are and share them with others. Fully own up to the power of your presence.

This book is about nourishing your cells, soul, skin, and spirit with a holistic inside-out approach. So, go on! Act like a queen with her crown on, strutting in style, standing tall. Walk with purpose while having a laid back, humble, happy presence, because that will be a power that you and others will feel instantly.

Connect four

As you gain a better sense of self-awareness and become more conscious, mindful, and wholesome, get to know these four factors that will help keep you aligned, connected, and beautifully balanced so that you truly thrive in all areas of life. These four factors are your physical, emotional, spiritual, and mental health.

When you start to pay attention, feel in tune with your body, and implement the f.a.b lifestyle tips, you will naturally boost, balance, and beautify yourself from inside out. Try to check in with yourself on a regular basis, make sure you feel that all four factors are getting equal attention.

When you wake up in the morning, approach the day with the end in mind. How do you want to feel by the end of the day? Accomplished? Healthy? Productive? Calm? Content? Or just simply happy?

Becoming aware and nourishing your physical, emotional, spiritual, and mental health will help naturally boost vitality and a sense of wellbeing for your body on all levels. Some people may feel there is one area that is more balanced than others. If you find that this is the case, simply infuse more energy into that part of your life.

For example, if you feel physically, emotionally, and mentally well, but your spirituality is suffering, spend some time in nature, or dedicate time for reflection, reiki, meditation, journaling, yoga, or simply being kind to yourself and others. I know for myself I have felt off in areas during times in my life, and over the years, practicing mindfulness, adopting a sense of awareness in my wellness regime, and really paying attention to imbalances help me spend more energy toward the parts of my life that need more love and care.

Master a fabulous mindset

For me food, fitness, and a fun-loving mindset are the foundation to feeling fu**ing fantastic. Your mindset requires lots of love and attention to your emotional, spiritual and mental health. Make a commitment to ditch judgment, self-doubt, struggles within yourself, bad vibes, and Debbie-downer behaviour. Shift your mindset and perspective to a fu**ing fabulous, upbeat one instead. Do this, and your outside world and reality will literally change.

I know this doesn't happen overnight. It does take time to train your brain to think the best, most fab, upbeat thoughts; however, as you work on flexing this muscle often, it will come naturally to you. You'll just feel good about feeling good, find small things to appreciate, and remember how blessed you and fortune you are.

Become the person you would admire and love. You know those people you meet that just are so comfortable in their own skin? The ones who are just real, and honest and truly nice, and clearly rock that fabulous mindset? They are confident and content with who they are. They embrace their strengths.

You deserve to live a fabulous life

This is a really important part of the fabulous formula. You must constantly remind yourself and truly believe that you deserve to live a fabulous life. You deserve to wake up every morning with a surge of energy that lights you up. You deserve to become the fabulous woman, or person, you should be. You deserve to be happy. You deserve to live a life you are excited about and proud of. You deserve the best. It is time to live your truth, and switch your self-doubting mind to a fabulous-thinking one from this day forward.

Creating and living a fabulous life starts with a choice. You must choose to live fabulously starting *today*, not tomorrow or next week or year. **Today**, say to yourself, "I deserve to feel fulfilled and live a fabulous life," and don't settle for anything less.

You truly deserve all the fabulous things life has to offer! Think fabulous, feel fabulous, live fabulous, and act fabulous. You will feel amazing and unstoppable when you realize you deserve to live in the fab lane. So cheers to a fabulous life! Go and celebrate with a glass of champagne with some of your best friends tonight! Just simply celebrate life.

Learn from the older and wiser

As I am touching on the topic in this part of "living fabulously," I thought I would end this section with some tips, tools, and good old wisdom from centenarians that all seemed to have similar advice about life.

Even though I try to live my life to the fullest, make the most of it, and not take it for granted after experiencing hardships and tough times, nothing is better than learning from those who have lived a full life already.

According to Bronnie Ware, author of "The Top Five Regrets of the Dying" of those who are nearing the end of their lives regret the following:

- Lacking courage to live life true to oneself
- Losing touch with friends
- Working excessively at the expense of familial companionship

- Lacking courage to express one's feelings
- Letting worries detract from happiness

Many centenarians also pointed out that close connections to loved ones, social interactions, and a sense of humor also were big factors in contributing to longevity and getting through harder times and health problems.

> **"The love of what you do, combined with your belief in what you do, will not determine your success. It will determine how hard you will work and how dedicated you will be to achieving it."**
>
> **– Jeffrey Gitomer**

In today's world, life can feel more stressful, hectic, or just simply out of balance. Your to-do lists might be getting longer, and time seems to disappear more quickly. Maybe your sense of well-being feels completely off.

It is not realistic to assume that life will mostly be smooth sailing. Tough times happen, financial problems may take a toll, or health issues could come up. Perhaps general real-life adulting forces you to take on responsibilities in many different areas of life.

Soak up new experiences, educate yourself, and read books on personal development, spirituality, health, and nutrition. Pursue your passions, follow your bliss, and do what makes you feel happy. Surround yourself with art and culture, do seasonal declutters to get rid of stuff that just doesn't bring any sparkle to your life anymore. Make an effort to be mindful of your thoughts, actions, and deeds towards yourself and others. Ditch judgement, and most importantly, make self-care a priority. Remember, self-care is not selfish — it is selfless.

> **"If your beliefs are limitless and ever evolving, your life will be too."**
>
> **—Unknown**

Overview for Living Fab

- Adopt a positive attitude and make an effort every day
- Follow your dreams and listen to your intuition
- Face your fears, and don't let fear become an option
- Surround yourself with art
- Pursue your passions
- Boost your brain beautifully with 20 minutes a day of inspirational reading.
- Believe in yourself, and your abilities, talents, and dreams.
- Make selfcare a priority
- Declutter your life
- Exude confidence in all areas of your life
- Stay present and be here now.
- Know that you deserve to live a fabulous life
- Joie de vivré i.e. a delight in being alive; keen, carefree enjoyment of living, literally, joy of living.)
- Become a life-lover and live fully
- Know that you are worthy of greatness
- Send out good, positive vibes — and get good vibes back

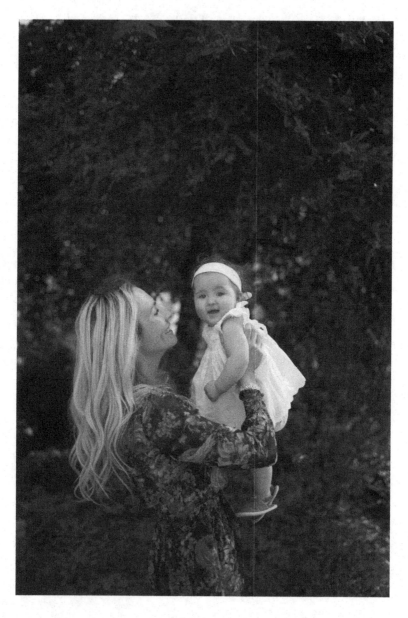

Motherhood is the most amazing, rewarding, challenging,
life changing thing that I am most proud of

PART 4

Look Fab

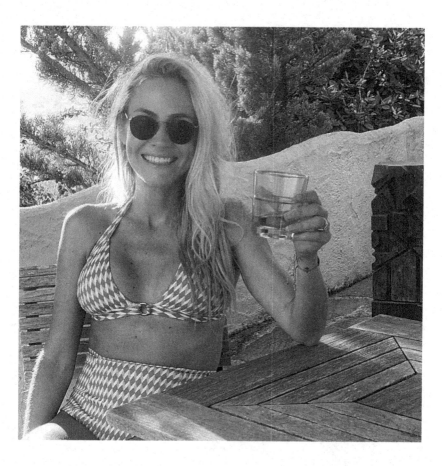

Keep your face to the sun and you will never see the shadows

Now that you have been eating real, wholesome foods, practicing positivity, expressing gratitude, striving to make joy your highest purpose, and learning to love your true, authentic self, we come to the final part of this guide: looking fab. The tips and tricks mentioned throughout the book will help boost, balance, and beautify your body, but I wanted to make the "physical" part of this book come last,

I believe it is important to first feed your mind and body with nourishing thoughts, affirmations, intentions, and foods to help rebalance yourself first, ridding the body of toxins both mentally and physically.

Striving to look great can sometimes have a negative spin on it. Some may even say it's vain, superficial, or selfish; however, my philosophy is that if you feel great, you look great, and if you look great, you feel great.

Think about a time, you got your hair done, put on some heels, and wore a figure-hugging dress. Did you not feel confident inside? Personally, if I have woken up bloated, blotchy, and have bad hair, my inner mood is definitely not the same as it is when my tummy is flat, my hair is fab, and my skin is glowing.

We all come in different shapes and sizes, but the key to a beautiful body is loving what you have, taking care of yourself, and embracing your best features, as well as eating well and enjoying activities that will burn fat and keep you trim and toned, no matter what shape you are.

Learn to love the body you have, and focus on beauty food feasting, rocking a positive attitude, loving yourself, and implementing daily movement, which definitely gives you physical benefits. Plus, once you switch to the beauty food mindset and find exercise that you love, you will feel a surge of energy, and motivation.

Here are my top tips to looking fab all the time.

"Health is not a mere absence of disease, it is an expression of life- in terms of how joyful, loving and enthusiastic you are."

—Sri Sri Ravi Shankar

Practice some form of movement every day

Moving your body, exercising, keeping fit, staying active, burning fat — whatever you want to call it — is an essential part of optimal health and wellbeing. It raises your heart rate, produces feel-good hormones, strengthens muscles, and helps us sweat out fat and toxins. I believe at least 150 minutes a week of proper physical activity is the key to looking healthy and strong on top of some form of daily movement.

Although I explored classes, like spin, boxing, body conditioning, personal training sessions, running, and general gym circuits, my top workouts that made me feel and see a difference were combining yoga, Pilates, and a bit of barre.

Yoga combines, breathing, moving, and meditation, while Pilates focuses on breathing, resistance training, and more challenging techniques focused around the core. The yoga-Pilates combination (or as I like to call it, "yogalates") got me long and lean, toned and tight, strong and slim, and happy and harmonious.

I believe mixing up strengthening, fat burning, and mental-building workouts will give you a whole holistic healthy fit package. Physical activity plays an important role in your health, well-being and quality of life.

Improve your health by being active as a part of a healthy lifestyle. Move your body every single day, even if it's just a brisk walk, and schedule a least 150 minutes a week of vigorous movement. Get into a routine and find a way to move your body every day. Find an exercise you love, a new class that sounds fun, or the latest fitness DVD or apps you can follow along with in the comfort of your own home. Mindful movement is crucial to the fabuloucity formula.

Either way, there is no excuse to not make the time for movement. Pencil it in and make the time. I prefer going in the a.m. to get it done and over with. Sometimes, I will go on my lunch break, as I like my evenings free; however, I may do one or two classes in the evenings now that I have a baby. Regardless, movement is a priority, so I make time for it. One hour of that ME time on my mat brings balance to my inner health.

Everyone is different, so find something that you love and your body loves. Treat classes like appointments. Schedule them in your diary and work your day-to-day living around it. There are 24 hours in a day, and 168 hours in a week. Penciling in four to five classes a week is manageable when you become organized. Check out local studios that offer these classes or if you have limited time, check out online workouts like Cody app, on YouTube, or a DVD, so you can do it in the comfort of your own home. Even as little as 30 minutes at home will give you major benefits.

When you move your body often and combine cardio, strength training, and stretching, you are bound to get your body long, lean, healthy and strong. You will melt fat, boost your metabolism, and not to mention, elevate your mood with a surge of endorphins. Make an effort to move every day, and get your heart rate up, even if you just take a brisk walk. If you live in a city where you drive everywhere, try to park farther away, and always take the stairs. Those extra steps really do make a difference.

Get Some Fresh Air

Make sure to get at least 15 minutes a day of a brisk walk and fresh air. Step out during your lunch, park your car further away, get off at an earlier train, tube, or subway stop. Or, do what I did and adopt a dog — you'll walk at least 30 minutes extra a day.

Walking has both physical and mental benefits. It increases your heart rate and gives you a nice glow for the day. Getting out and surrounding yourself with nature is so healing and refreshing. Stop and smell the flowers, pause and gaze at the green plants, or look up at the snowflakes falling. Be grateful in those minutes of being outside.

So many people who don't live in sunny conditions all year long are extremely deficient in vitamin D, so on top of eating D-rich foods like fish, nuts, seeds, and mushrooms, take a supplement and make sure to get outside every day.

Go Glam, Girl

Get up, dress up, and show up. Whether you work in the corporate world and have a certain attire or are a freelancer and work in activewear, keeping your mane tame, nails neat, and face polished will automatically get you into a motivated mindset.

While appearance is not the most important aspect of my fabulosity formula, it makes up a fraction of it. Having good grooming habits is just as important as diet and lifestyle ones.

Let's face it: when you look good, you feel good.

No matter what, I make time for my hair to be blown out, as well as a nail appointment each week. I always put on a bit of tinted moisturizer and lip gloss for an instant pick-me-up. Having good hair, polished nails, and a fresh face will boost your confidence instantly. As you become the most fab version of you, your confidence should grow by the day.

Looking good will lift you up, as well as boost your mood, give you confidence and motivation. It might sound shallow, but image and first impressions do play a big part in our society. Think about when you have come across someone with sloppy clothes, messy hair, and chipped nails — you might not have had the best impression of them.

Budget or no budget, make time for self-care, make an effort to look your best every day, have nice hair, keep your nails neat, and put on some lip gloss — you never who you may bump into, and if you don't get out much, make effort for yourself. It will make you feel better and give you a gentle reminder of how beautiful you are. Make the most of your best attributes, and love what you have. Learn to play around with natural yet glowing goddess looks.

"I believe that all women are pretty without makeup — but the right makeup can be pretty powerful"

—Bobbi brown.

"When you are glowing and feel great, your confidence will soar."

—Ashley Siedentopf

Style and Dressing Up

As a former stylist and fashion student in London and Milan, I have a decent amount of knowledge in the fashion sector. Even as a young girl, my grandparents would take care of me on weekends, where I would choose to start our Saturdays with a shopping trip to the mall (which makes me giggle) or carefully plan out my outfits the night before school in elementary and middle school. I would get my inspiration from magazines like Teen Vogue, Seventeen, and Cosmo.

During my pre-teen years, I would even give my friends head-to-toe makeovers. There was something about transforming someone's image to make them look amazing that gave me such a buzz. Feeling and looking good go hand-in-hand, as discussed in previous chapters, so style is the last part of my fabulosity formula.

"Style is a way to say who you are without having to speak."

— celebrity stylist, Rachel Zoe

I couldn't agree more with this quote. Even if you have a strict budget, high-street shops now have amazing pieces that are on-trend without the hefty price tag. Having spent a fair amount of time in Paris and previously worked as a personal stylist, something I noticed was the French women's sense of style. It was effortless, timeless, undone, and utterly cool. No matter what is trendy at the moment, the pieces I used to tell clients to invest in and still would today are:

- Chic trench coat
- Good pair of fitted, black jeans
- Leather, or faux leather, pants
- Great pair of dark-blue fitted jeans
- High-quality leather jacket
- Classic snug-fitting black dress
- Simple white cotton T-shirt
- Pair of black pointed high heel pumps
- Jean jacket
- Sexy, colourful pair of strappy sandals
- Pair of flat biker boots
- Pair of chic ballerina slippers
- Comfy a pair of white or black sneakers, and you can never go wrong with adding cute jewellery for accessories.

If you need some extra inspiration in the style department, go out and purchase the latest fashion magazines for some inspiration, or hire a personal stylist.

If you are investing in your wardrobe, this is a great time to get rid of old, unwearable, outdated clothes! Or as they say, "Out the with old, in the with new." Go through every item and ask yourself, "Do I LOVE this? Is it in good condition? Does it spark lots of happiness? Is it going to make me look fab or drab?"

As you are transforming yourself from the inside out, there is no better time to give yourself a fresh new look or simply just treat yourself to a few new key pieces that you can mix and match. Looking good instantly makes you feel good. When you make the extra effort to put together a cute outfit, it not only gets your creative juices flowing, but gives you a natural boost of confidence.

If you love rocking all black, try adding a pop of red lip gloss with some gold accessories, or maybe wear a bold-print colorful dress and cute chunky boots.

Fashion should be fun. It is a way to express yourself and make you feel good. Your sense of style and clothes will affect your mood, confidence, and spirit. You don't need to be all flashy and go all O.T.T to communicate and express to the world who you are; although for makeup, I'm all about less is more. However, when it comes to clothes, the world is your oyster. Think chunky knits with leather leggings and boots, a long print dress and colorful heels, boyfriend jeans with a cute jumper, or a statement tee with a bold print skirt. There are so many fun ways you can play with fashion, and you can still do it all on a budget, so go grab some fashion magazines on a sunny afternoon, get some inspiration. Then, plan a date to shop.

"No matter how you feel, get up, dress up, show up, and never give up."

Unknown

Glowing, gorgeous skin makes all the difference

Having a clear, glowing complexion is the first sign of looking healthy, youthful, and vibrant no matter what age you are. Beautiful, glowing skin is always your best beauty accessory. I am a firm believer that gorgeous skin starts from within, so by making beauty food feasting a part of your daily lifestyle, your skin will benefit tremendously.

It is also important to have a beauty routine to maximize the benefits of high-quality nutrition. It is vital to keep your skin protected, hydrated, and nourished from a topical point. Since my early teens I have loved buying new beauty products that make me feel good. I believe that taking care of your skin is a form of self-love and self-care.

The essential things you need are a good simple cleanser, exfoliator, toner, sunscreen, day/night crème, serum, and facial oil. I cannot particularly recommend a brand as there are so many amazing ones on the markets these days; however, my best advice is to do some research on a few that seem to be the most popular and book a consultation with the beauty advisor to have them recommend the best products for your skin type. I love scheduling a facial when I have time, but what I really enjoy is doing weekly at-home beauty treatments a couple of times a week, implementing extra masks, moisturizers, face massages, serums, and facial oils for added hydrating, nourishing, purifying, and radiating benefits. Plus, the idea of pampering one to two times a week is a form of self-love, which combines both skincare and self-care in the comfort of my own home. It's a win-win scenario, I say.

It is important to cleanse, scrub, treat, tone, nourish and protect, so look for a brand you love that is gentle on your skin. Don't go to bed with your makeup on ever. This is a huge No-No. Dirty skin leads to dull and damaged skin, so no matter how many drinks you may have had or how burned out you may feel, wash your face at night. Keep your facial wipes next to your bed in case you have a late night or feel exhausted.

Although I love spending time in the sun, I cover up with high SPF protection and always make sure to wear a big hat and sunglasses, and I try to be near shade, so I have extra coverage on my face. No matter how much botching and botox you think you can do, too much sun exposure, smoking, and a diet of processed foods will damage and age your Always use high SPF sunscreen protection and wear hats and shades when you're in sunny climates, and feast on beauty foods.

Skincare Routine for Glowing Skin

- **Cleanser:** In the morning, go for a gentle cleansing micellar water. There are some combined products that both cleanse and tone. In the evening, use a more gel-based or cleansing balm-type of product to remove dirt, impurities, and makeup.
- **Scrub:** Exfoliate two to three times per week before cleansing to remove dead skin cells and boost natural radiance.
- **Tone:** After your daily cleansing, use a toner to balance out the skin and texture. You can also find micellar cleansers now that also tone for convenience.
- **Sleep Serum:** Apply a serum in the evening over your moisturizer to nourish, repair and protect your skin, while helping lift away dead skin cells for better skin texture, reduction of prominent wrinkles, and a luminous canvas.
- **Organic Facial Oils:** These oils are ultra-nourishing, moisturizing, and age-defying. Use them one to two times per day over your moisturizer.
- **Vitamin C Serum:** Use this serum to brighten, lift, and firm. Vitamin C serum gives you that glow factor, so use it in the morning under your moisturizer, and facial oil.
- **Protection:** wear a UVB sunscreen, even if you don't live in a super sunny place. You could even use a tinted moisturizer that gives you protection plus light coverage.
- **Moisturizer:** Apply a light moisturizer in the morning and a rich moisturizer at night before your serum and facial oil.
- **Hydrate:** Spritz your skin with a face mist to hydrate and nourish. And of course, sip on at least eight glasses of mineral water a day.
- **Weekly face masks** for maximum glow boosting benefits

Load up on skin-loving ingredients

Beauty food feasting definitely has a positive impact on the appearance of your skin, as it is focused on natural nutrition, which is nourishing, healing, anti- inflammatory, and beautifying. However, there are some skin-loving foods with extra beauty-boosting properties, that help with radiance, texture, and plumpness from within.

Foods rich in antioxidants A, C, and E, and omega 3s are great for your skin. Stock up on leafy greens, berries, wild fish, avocado, nuts, eggs, seeds, bone broths, supplements, and superfoods.

<u>Ashfab Skin-Loving Care tip</u>

Try to set aside 20 to 30 minutes one to two times per week for the ultimate home beauty treatment while you take a bath, meditate, or for me, both. :-)

Start with a gentle cleanser. Exfoliate and apply a toner, followed by your favorite face mask. Then massage your face with one or two types of facial oils, and finish off with your serum and night cream.

By massaging oils two to three times per week onto your skin, you are actually implementing Abhyanga into your wellness routine, Abhyanga derives from the ancient Indian Ayurvedic self-treatment traditions. By adding Abhyanga practice to your self-care regime, you are naturally restoring the balance in your body while enhancing your wellbeing and beauty. Regular Abhyanga is grounding and relaxing, leaving you with a deep feeling of warmth, strength, and stability. This gives you a mega dose of skincare, self-care, and self-love.

Soon I will be launching Ashí Belle Organics, an at home botanical beauty ritual range, a topical skin nutrition that combines skin care and self care in one, set along with other beauty, bath and body care products i.e. nutrition for your skin. It will be available online soon since getting regular facials is not always accessible. Doing them at home instead is both effective and affordable.

It's all about attitude

Do you remember a time when you met a super pretty person, but as soon as they spoke, and you observed their body language, all you could see was a bad attitude and bad vibes, and it just made them not-so-pretty anymore?

This is because attitude is one of the first things you notice about a person. When you meet someone kind, cool, down-to-Earth, and warm, you will remember them positively, right? On the other hand, someone with an arrogant, egotistical attitude may not leave that nice feeling, because first impressions make a huge impact, both good and bad. As you become more mindful, aware of your thoughts, actions, beliefs, and feelings, and simply more in tune with yourself, bear in mind, the attitude you bring to the table will be the impression you leave when you meet someone new.

The "Wow" Factor

Having the wow factor is not just about being born a super model with long legs and a small waist; having the wow factor is truly an inside-out-approach. We are all born unique, and beautiful in our own right. With proper nutrition, we not only feel good, but we can delay or slow down the signs of aging and look glowing and healthy. When you think pretty thoughts, act kindly, and do good deeds for others, your beauty will radiate out of you like rays of sunshine.

Shifting a pessimistic mindset to an optimistic attitude will boost endorphins and serotonin, which send good vibes from the inside out. Moving your body daily by finding a fitness class you like will get you strong, sculpted, long, and lean. Plus, it will give you another sense of purpose. Stand tall, walk with confidence, and rock that wow factor — we all have it within us. You've just got to unleash it.

When you nourish your body with vibrant foods, you will feel a shift of energy, have a better mood, and really feel fantastic. Opening your mindset to loving, positive, grateful, happy thoughts will do wonders for your wow factor too. Living in the present, doing what you love, practicing self-care and self-love, and being mindful of your thoughts, feelings, actions, and emotions will propel you to vibrant health, It will bring out your natural beauty from within. So rock that wow factor, and remember we all have it within us!

"Invest in your skin; it's going to represent you for a long time."

Unknown

Looking fab is the last part of the f.a.b formula. By nourishing your mind, body, soul, and spirit with healthy mantras, mat workouts, and meals based on beauty food feasting, you can turbo-boost your health and feel energetic, positive, and happy. Not to mention, you'll be healthy and strong while looking well and glowing from the inside-out.

Make the effort to move your body, invest in your skin, and take care of it daily. Set aside some time for self-care with an at-home skin pampering session each week. Put on a little make up every day, fix up your hair, keep your nails neat, and you will feel like a million bucks in no time! It truly goes hand-in-hand; when you look great, you feel great, and vice versa. All of these tips are actually forms of self-care, so you are essentially boosting your inner self love battery at the same time.

Overview:

- Move your body every single day, even just for 30 minutes. Do at least 150 minutes a week of dynamic moments. Find something you love, do it well and often
- Declutter your wardrobe, invest in some timeless pieces, and find a style that suits your personality and mood
- Look groomed. Good hair, polished nails, and a little lip gloss will help your confidence go from zero to hero.
- Natural beauty shines and radiates from within, and glowing skin is your best accessory, so take care of it. Focus on beauty food feasting for skin loving benefits and get plenty of sleep or rest when you an if you have kids
- Have a daily skincare regime. Implement Abhyanga one to two times per week and invest in your skin.

- Get out for fresh air daily. It will clear your head and boost your mood daily, while helping the blood flow for a natural skin glow
- Watch out for my Ashí Belle Organics line; a topical skin nutrition range which will include at home a 5 step weekly facial set, daily maintenance facial oils, essential oils, candles, crystal facial rollers, and bath, chakra gem sets body and baby care

Ashfab Lifestyle

I am mindful of my thoughts and actions. I meditate daily. I move daily. I connect with loved ones often. I practice yoga. I fill my plates with plants and natural nutrition. I make self-care and self-love a priority so that I can feel my best and put 100 percent into all other areas of my life. I can have bad days too, just like anybody else, but I always start my day and go to bed with a grateful heart. I remember I am alive: I have food to eat, a warm house, supportive friends and family, clothes to wear, and clean water to drink, so by simply focusing on all the good things I have in my life, I create an abundance.

Life is precious. We only have one, and I believe that we should make every day count. We should value each day as if it were our last. We should nourish ourselves with the best foods to feel better, live longer, and look younger, and we should never stop dancing, laughing, or having fun no matter what age we are.

There is always room for improvement to upgrade ourselves and our lives right now. We must check in with ourselves and figure out what is not working and what is working. We must infuse energy and extra love in areas of our lives that need improvement, from career, money, relationships, home life, spirituality, exercise, creativity, and self-care.

Without thinking about what if, or "I can't because of so and so," write down what you would like your life to look like. What do you want to do? What do you want to achieve? Where do you want to live? Who is in your life? How do you feel? How do you look? How is your health? Do you travel?

Remember, no matter where you are, you can be and do anything you put your mind to! I still have so many steps to climb before I reach the top; however, when I look back at where I was and how far I have come, I am truly grateful for my past, the present moment, and what my future will entail.

I am sitting here right now writing this book to inspire and empower others about feeling and looking fabulous from the inside out, which makes me happy because I am speaking from the heart and sharing my message with fellow females and other readers. The best project you can ever work on is yourself, physically, mentally, spiritually, and intellectually. Nourish your mind, body, soul, and spirit with the best things, foods, thoughts, and movement. Surround yourself with uplifting, positive, happy people.

Connect with Mother Earth, and enjoy nature. Listen to music, step out of your comfort zone, and do something that scares you. Remove fear, doubt, and negative vibes from your life; these are harmful to both inner and outer health. Holistic healing revolves around your mind, body, spirit, and emotions — in the quest for optimal health and wellness, on top of supplementation, meditation, yoga, reiki, acupuncture, massages, mindfulness, journaling, and homeopathic remedies, all help boost, balance and beautify you from the inside out.

The more sense of awareness you have within yourself, the more in tune you become with imbalances, like aches, pains, struggles, stress, and low moods. So as we come to the end of the book, make yourself your number ONE priority. Make a commitment to work on Project YOU.

My book contains a wealth of tips to help you turbo-boost your health, wellbeing, and beauty. So dream big, live large, imagine a beautiful life, vibrant health, so much love, laughs, and fun times, because our thoughts are the powerhouse to our reality. If you have always had a low-vibing, pessimistic, procrastinating, poor way of thinking, you will get the same negative energy in return. So you might as well opt for joy, love, and happy emotions as these are what will propel your growth as a person.

Healing occurs when we become something better than what we were before, so regardless, working on and taking care of ourselves is a life-long commitment and journey. You will only feel better along the way.

If you have never done any type of work on yourself and you always put self-care at the bottom of your to-do list, don't be stunned if you feel worse before you feel better. Just like removing harmful foods and adding in good ones, detoxing from harmful thoughts, actions, and beliefs is a form of detoxification, so think of this as a protocol to vibrant health, wellness, and natural beauty.

As I share these tricks, tips, and tools that I have learned from my own healing journey over the past 25 years, remember healing does not happen overnight. It takes time and requires discipline, dedication, devotion, hard work, patience, positivity, and self-belief.

By making a commitment to eat the most fabulous foods, think and affirm fabulous thoughts about yourself, do and experience fabulous things, surround yourself with fabulous people, get fabulously fit, and make an effort to look fabulous every day, then I have no doubt you will feel and look fabulous from the inside out.

If you become obsessive with calorie counting and eating clean daily, it will cause imbalance. Don't overdo it. Simply eat natural nutrition, treat yourself when you need to, and find a happy balance for your wellbeing, beauty, and body. Nourishing yourself with affirmations, meditation, positive thoughts, visualisation, journaling, mindfulness, inspirational reading, motivational podcasts, and creating, and connecting with loved ones, is so important for our mental, emotional and spiritual health.

The great thing about my Fab living approach is that there is no one-size-fits-all. By addressing your health concerns, imbalances, modifying your diet, adding supplements, and taking time off to reconnect with yourself, will help combat accelerated ageing, lifestyle-related illnesses, chronic pain, and weight gain, as well as improve your mood and memory by boosting your body to a balanced state from the inside out.

I hope my tips, tricks, tools and recipes are helpful to you. You can use them for yourself and share with loved ones around you too. Having our health is truly our greatest wealth; without it, we have nothing. So put you and your health first, and don't ever be hard on yourself. Be patient, persistent, and stay positive on your new path to fabulosity, because you deserve it! I hope you will feel inspired to want to eat, feel, live, and look your most fab self now. It's never too late to start a new way of living that brings out the best in you.

Here's to feeling and looking fabulous, because life is for living, and it should be lived in a fabulous way from the inside out starting today! Cheers to the fab life. Now go and celebrate the new you — with some champagne of course. ;-)

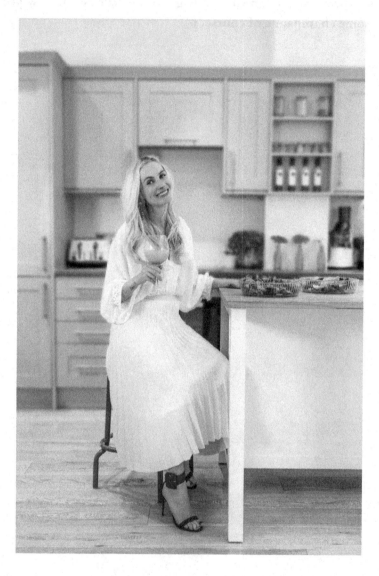

5.5 months pregnant here and I was already so in love with Lula Belle before I had met her

ASHFAB LIFESTYLE
IN A NUTSHELL

- Implement the daily ritual of drinking the 3 age defying blends
- *Start your mornings off with a beauty elixir shot*
- *Sip on a nutrient-packed, plant-based smoothie for breakfast*
- *Drink a large, cold-pressed veggie juice daily, and sip 8–9 glasses of purified, water per day for hydration*
- Eat off of smaller plates. Take small bites, and chew well so that your body can digest your food properly
- Take superfoods and supplements for optimal cellular health
- Read 20 minutes of something uplifting, inspirational, or motivating every day. It will keep your mind young, and give your brain a good workout — not to mention, you might read some advice that will change your life for the better.
- Move your body with effective exercise for at least 20 minutes daily and 150 minutes a week of dynamic movement. Find classes you love and walk as much as you can. Improve your strength and flexibility, and get your heart rate up often. Mix up your workouts. You deserve a strong, healthy body
- Add regular holistic style therapies like reiki, acupuncture, deep tissue and lymphatic massages for extra love and care for a deep sense of wellbeing
- Meditate daily for 20 minutes and practice mindfulness
- Include plants at all meals and aim for 7–9 servings of fruit, berries, leafy greens, and veggies through wellness shots, smoothies, soups, sides, salads and fresh juices. Plan your meal around plants, and

make other stuff the sides and condiments. Simply add in lots of good sh** to crowd out the bad

- Focus on high vibe living, when you become more self aware and mindful, you will notice when bad vibes are setting in, so zap it and go back to happy vibes
- Release negative thoughts, beliefs, and self-limitations. Switch to positive ones. When times are tough, try to look for the sunshine and brightness around you. There is always light at the end of the tunnel
- Everything will be ok, so have hope and faith in the future
- Simply think, act, speak, and feel with a loving heart, and lead your life with love. You will experience joy and appreciation rather than resentment, anger or jealousy
- Affirm what you want, not what you don't want in life. Your thoughts create your reality — literally. Uplifting mantras, positive mental imagery, and visualization of dreams and desires are extremely powerful and will help you create the life you want
- Express 3–5 things you are grateful for, and count your blessings in the morning and before bed. A grateful heart is the gateway to true abundance in all areas of your life
- Maintain great hair, nice nails, and enhance your best features in a natural way with light makeup (less is more). Take care of your skin. Make an effort to look groomed and gorgeous, even if it's not a special occasion. Carry yourself with all the confidence in the world — you deserve it!
- Love yourself so much. Be your own best friend. Ditch judgmental, critical thoughts, negative self-talk, and never doubt your ability to be fabulous and amazing. Breathe in compassion, breath out criticism

- Make time for laughter. Don't take yourself so seriously. Lighten up and have a sense of humor. Humor allows us to have positive feelings of joy and amusement in any situation
- Trust the process, be patient with the present, be grateful of your journey, and believe in yourself. Live fully every day, shine bright from within, love your life, and life will love you right back!

The End

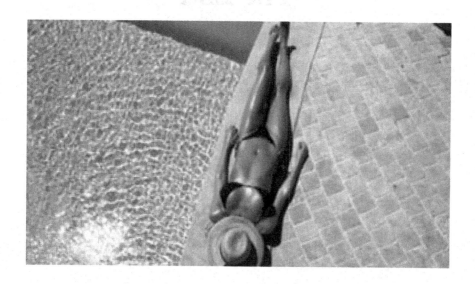

Be grateful of your journey

ACKNOWLEDGMENTS

This book would not have been possible without my husband Topper — my rock, my soul mate, and the biggest supporter of my growth and career. He believed in me, had faith in me, always stood behind me, lifted me up when things were tough, and reminded me to keep going. Because of his relentless love and support, we have grown together on this journey. I am truly grateful for his self-healing, progression, and efforts to understand my passion for health, spirituality, nutrition, mindfulness, meditation, holistic therapies, and so on. More than an amazing husband, he's been a wonderful student, and his eagerness to learn throughout this process has helped me become the teacher that I am meant to be in this world. He went through his own struggle and battled some inner demons half way through this book, which had tested our relationship however with hope, faith and belief, he found the light and has continued to be on his own type of healing journey.

I would also like to express my utmost gratitude for my parents, who were there for me twenty-four-seven, from my diagnosis early in childhood and thereafter. Now that I have a daughter of my own, I can't even begin to imagine the stress and despair my diagnosis must have caused my whole family. I am forever grateful, particularly toward my mother — whom I cannot thank enough — for her determination to find better ways to heal me holistically, even in the 90's when the internet resources we have now were not so readily available. Her guidance taught me so much about natural health, since our doctors at the time only believed in pills and potions and eating the standard American diet.

I also want to send my love to both my sister and brother, Kate and Tristan, whom I love, love, LOVE so much. I have missed them so much over the years, but soon, I hope, I will be closer, just a short flight away, so we can make up for lost times.

And who could forget Magnus, the first person I connected with when I left Canada for Europe? We've been roommates in Milan and London, witnessed each other's marriages, danced on tables together, gone through breakups, sipped way too many martinis, and worked together in fashion — we've basically seen it all! We've grown together since 2004, and while we may be on totally different paths, I am so grateful for our special bond we have and the uncontrollable giggles we have in the wrong moments lol...Since 2004, we've spoken to each other everyday, and I hope we always will.

To the people around the world who stood by me, my nearest and dearest soul sistas, my besties, I'd like to say thank you! They were always there for me, they believed in me and inspired me, and they never competed with me or judged me. They made me laugh, loved me for me, and supported me all the way. They know who they are, a big Shout-out to London, NYC, Brazil, L.A, Toronto, and Edmonton.

Uncle Mikey, the older brother I never had, I'd like to thank for all his love, support, and kindness over the years. He is the kindest, most sincere person who never expects, wants, or asks for anything in return, except for everyone to be happy. I wish him all the happiness he deserves, and for all the people he is there for, too!

I'd like to thank my grandma in the U.K. who taught me the importance of kindness, sharing, and being nice to everyone — not to mention, reading, writing, telling time, and tying my shoelaces. I spent a fair amount of time in the U.K., from the age of 6-weeks-old to Kindergarten, and afterward, I returned in the summertime. A taste of British upbringing, including being polite and having good manners, really helped shape who I am today.

It is said that in the first seven years of your life, the relationships you have, how you are raised, and the experiences you endure both good and bad, have a profound impact on the person you become. For that, I'd like to mention my nana and papa, whom I spent countless weekends with when they lived nearby. I have so many fond memories with them, and although they really did spoil me with presents, what they spoiled me with most was their presence and the lovely attention and affection they gave me, which has had a tremendously positive effect on how I freely, confidently show love to others today. As they say, "You can still think you're amazing and fabulous without thinking you're better than others."

Finally, I would like to thank my extended family, especially my father in law, who was the sweetest, kindest man. He always took an interest in my wellness journey, and he gave me great compliments and positive feedback on my work, which meant so much to me. He will forever be in our hearts and never forgotten.

Recipes for Radiant skin and vibrant health

Natural, nourishing dishes to help boost, balance and beautify from the inside out! These Fabulous feasts that are bursting with fresh produce, fun flavour and just the right amount of protein. Nutritious and delicious meals made in minutes. Feel good foods to make you feel and look fabulous from the inside out!

Recipes for radiant skin, vibrant health, and loads of energy.

#Fabfoodfeasting

Nutritious and delicious plant based meals made in minutes

- *Soups:* Soups are a fabulous option nutritionally as they combine key nutrients, including vitamins, minerals, that are nutrient dense; meaning high in nutrients but low in calories, while still keeping you satisfied. Get pure comfort in delicious recipes that make great meals at any time of the day
- *Salads:* - Sumptuous salads bursting with vitamins, minerals, and antioxidants are the perfect way to get your daily dose of essentials, in just one bowl.
- *Savory suppers:* These fabulous feasts are bursting with fresh produce, fun flavour, and just the right amount of plant based protein. Easy and enjoyable to make in minutes. Wow your friends or loved ones.
- *Smoothies* - Adding fresh smoothies to your daily routine is the quickest, and most effective way to get absorbed into your system

fast. Over you time you will feel a difference, see a difference and be a whole new you. plant based protein

- *Sweet treats* - simple sweet desserts: This collection of sweet greats are a combination of healthy and delicious ingredients. Satisfying enough to fill that craving.
- *Salad dressings* sexy salad dressings full of beautifying benefits
- *Beauty bowls:* a selection of sweet and savoury gluten grain based bowls that give you the perfect balance of healthy fat, plant protein and dietary fibre, to energise, curb cravings, satisfy for hours, packed with plethora of nutrients.

The servings sizes are indicated as 2-4 servings because they can be two generous portions or 4 small portions.

Salads

These sumptuous salads are bursting with vitamins, minerals and antioxidants, and are the perfect way to get your daily dose of your essentials in just one bowl. These nutrient packed salads will fill you up for hours, while being kind to your waistline.

Glowing gorgeous greens
Plant based beauty babe
Kale apple and walnut salad
Spicy asian love
Sexy Caesar salad

1) Glowing gorgeous goddess greens

Serve 2 - 4

Ingredients

- 2 cups of leafy greens of your choice
- 1 Cucumber chopped
- 1 Green pepper chopped
- 2 Tbsp of pumpkin seeds

- 2 Tbsp of crushed hazelnuts
- 1 Peeled Avocado chopped in cubes
- 1 cup of chopped mango

Optional Serve with

* 2 boiled free range eggs or wild caught salmon

Dressing

- 2 Tbsp of extra virgin oil
- 1/2 cup of purified water
- Juice of 1 lemon
- 1/4 goji berries
- 2 tbsp of Nutritional yeast flakes
- 1 tbsp of Tamari sauce
- 2 tbsp of raw honey
- Place dressing ingredients in blender in blender, blitz/ blend
- In a small bowl place the dressing ingredients and give a little whisk
- In a large bowl add the other ingredients and pour and toss the dressing
- **Tip:** if you need extra protein, add sautéed mushrooms, tofu or wild caught fish.

2) **Plant based beauty**

- 2 cups of de-stemmed spinach
- 1/2 cup of blueberries
- 1/2 cup of black berries
- 1 red pepper chopped
- 1 green pepper chopped
- 1/4 of poppy seeds

Dressing

1/2 cup of fresh lemon juice

1/4 Cup of flax oil

1/4 cup of Tahini

2 Tbsp of raw honey

2 Tsp of minced garlic

Instructions:

- Place dressing ingredients in blender in blender, blitz/ blend
- In a small bowl place the dressing ingredients and give a little whisk
- In a large bowl add the other ingredients and pour and toss the dressing
- Add the tofu last and serve immediately, enjoy!

3) **Kale, apple and walnut salad**

- 2 Cups of shredded kale, (soak for 10 minutes in salted water to soften)
- 1/2 chopped cucumber
- 1 tbs of chia seeds
- 2 Chopped apples
- 1 cup of walnuts
- 1/2 cup of goji berries

Dressing

- 1 tsp of dijon mustard
- 1 tbsp raw honey
- 1 tbsp of balsamic vinegar
- 2 tbsp of extra virgin oil

Instructions:

- Toast the walnuts for 10 minutes in preheated oven around 180 degrees
- In a small bowl whisk the dressing ingredients together

- Add the rest of the ingredients in a salad bowl, add the dressing and toss evenly.
- Sprinkle with chia seeds and walnuts

4) *Spicy asian love*

- 2 small bunches of broccoli chopped
- 1 small bunch of chopped asparagus
- 1 small bunch of trimmed, and halved green beans
- 1 packet of vermicelli rice noodles cooked as directed on the box.
- Sprinkle of sea salt and black pepper
- Sprinkle of crushed peanuts
- 2 Tsp of minced garlic
- Drizzle of hot sauce

Dressing

- 2 tsp of tamari gluten free soya sauce
- Drizzle of pure maple syrup
- 1 tsp of grated ginger
- 2 tbsp of sesame seeds
- 1 Tbsp of fresh orange juice

Optional" add your favourite plant protein or palm sized organic lean protein kick

Instructions:

- Boil water, and cook vermicelli noodles as directed meanwhile
- In a pan heat 1 tbsp of coconut oil, until melted and slightly sauté/ heat the vegetables until slightly golden (never overcook), next adding the garlic, salt, and pepper.
- Whisk the dressing ingredients together
- In 2 bowls, add the equal amount of noodles, then add your protein, lastly with the dressing.

5) Caesar Salad

Ingredients:

- 2 cups of washed and chopped leafy greens
- 2 tablespoons extra virgin olive oil
- 1/4 cup of Water
- 2 tablespoons Nutritional Yeast
- Sprinkle Sea salt and pepper to taste
- Coconut bacon (in a small pan heat 1/2 tbsp of coconut oil, 1/2 cup of coconut flakes, splash of tamari sauce, drizzle of maple syrup.
- Gluten free bread broken into cubes placed in the oven and drizzle with olive oil, sea salt, black pepper, garlic, and toast until golden around 10/ 15 minutes.
- 1 cup of chopped cherry tomatoes
- 1 cucumber sliced in half moons shapes

Dressing

- Juice from 1 lemon
- 1/2 cup raw cashews soaked overnight or in warm water for a10 minutes before to soften them.
- 2 tablespoons extra virgin olive oil
- 1/4 cup of Water a little more if needed in the food processor
- 1/2 tablespoons of minced garlic
- 2 tablespoons Nutritional Yeast
- Sprinkle Sea salt and pepper to taste

Soups: Sumptuous soups are a fabulous option nutritionally as they combine key nutrients, including vitamins, minerals, that are nutrient dense; meaning high in nutrients but low in calories, while still keeping you satisfied. Get pure comfort in delicious recipes that make great meals at any time of the day.

Vegetable garden
Butternut squash and carrot
Roasted creamy tomato soup

**Magical mushroom
Beauty broth**

1) Vegetable garden

- 250 ml of gluten free vegetable broth
- 1 can of canned chopped tomatoes
- 1 tube of tomato paste
- Small onion chopped
- 1 can of cannellini beans
- 2 Carrots chopped
- 1 courgette sliced in half moons
- 1 can of organic chick peas
- 1/2 tbsp of minced garlic
- Sea salt and ground black pepper to flavour
- 2 cups of cooked whole grain rice gluten free penne pasta

Instructions:

- Chop all the veg, cook the pasta while your doing that, cook pasta according to instructions make sure not to over cook set a timer on your phone,
- Add the broth, veg and pasta to a big post and simmer, cook on low constantly checking, for 45 min - 1 hour,
- Grate some vegan cheese or sheep milk cheese on top or serve with your favourite whole grain gluten free bread.

2) Butternut squash and carrot

- 250 ml of vegetable broth
- 1 cup of chopped butternut squash
- 1 cup of sweet potato chopped
- 4 carrots chopped
- 1 small onion chopped
- 1 -2 tbsp of minced garlic adjust to your taste buds
- 1/2 cup of soaked cashews (over night or in warm water for 10 minutes)

- Sea salt, ground black pepper
- Sprinkle of chilli flakes
- 1 small can of coconut creme
- very small amount of grated ginger just enough to flavour
- 1 tbsp of coconut oil

Instructions

- In a big pan, heat the coconut oil, add all the vegetable ingredients, and slightly heat for a few minutes to soften
- Next add to a food processor, then the remaining ingredients, blend for 5 minutes until smooth and heated, or if yours does not heat, pour into a bot and heat until warm, try not to let boil, Enjoy and serve hot.
- Finish off with a drizzle with some coconut creme.

3) <u>Roasted creamy tomato soup</u>

- 8 Roma tomatoes
- 1 tube of pure tomato paste
- 1 can of chopped tomatoes
- 250 ml of vegetable stock
- 1/2 cup of cashews soaked before.
- Drizzle of coconut creme
- 2 tsp of minced garlic
- 1/2 a small onion
- Sea salt and ground black pepper

Instructions:

Preheat the oven to 180 degrees, cover the baking tray with foil, and add the roma tomatoes, chopped onion, garlic, sea salt, ground black pepper, small onion, for 15 minutes. Next at the slightly cooked tomatoes to blender and add the remaining ingredients. Blend for 5 minutes until smooth.

4) **Magical mushroom soup**

- 1 tbsp of vegan butter
- Small onion chopped
- 250 ml of vegetable stock
- 2 packages of button mushrooms
- 1 small potato (pre boiled) and then sliced.
- 1 small can of coconut creme
- 2 tsp of minced garlic
- Sea salt and ground black pepper to taste.

Instructions:

- In a pan heat the vegan butter and onion until slightly golden brown than add the chopped mushrooms, garlic, sea salt and ground pepper, until mushrooms slightly cooked, next add to your food processor with the remaining ingredients, blend for 5 minutes or until smooth, serve immediately or if not heated transfer to a pot and heat until hot.

5) **Beauty broth** this recipe is gut healing, immune strengthening, skin loving, and a potent anti-inflammatory.

- 12 cups of mineral water *never tap water
- 2 tbsp avocado oil or olive oil
- 1 small/medium onion quartered
- 3 tsp of minced garlic
- Very small amount of grated ginger
- 3 cups of leafy greens like kale and spinach
- 5 Carrots
- 5 celery sticks
- Ground pepper and sea salt for taste
- 2 tbsp ground turmeric
- A bunch of fresh parsley
- 1/3 cup nutritional yeast flakes.

Instructions

- Add all the ingredients to a large pot. Heat on high to boil, then simmer, with the lid on, for an hour.
- After the hour, strain the liquid into a large bowl, than back in the large pot and simmer
- Serve immediately with some fresh herbs, for decoration or store in glass jars to have later on. It also freezes well.

Fabulous feasts

Pure love tomato penne
Spaghetti delight
Casserole love
Tacos
Asian stir-fry

1) Pure love tomato penne

Ingredients

- 2 cups of whole grain brown rice penne
- 1 tube of tomato paste
- 1 can of organic chopped tomatoes
- 1 cup of cherry tomatoes cut in half
- 1/2 a small jar of sun dried tomatoes
- Sprinkle of chilli flakes
- 1 tsp of olive oil
- Sea salt and ground black pepper
- 2 tsp of minced garlic

Instructions

- Cook pasta as directed and set aside (I always run some cold water over the pasta when drain it in the strainer, and also cooking gluten free pasta to perfection requires, not over or under cooking, so it tastes good, make sure water is boiled, and boil between 8-10 minutes with olive oil in water, and some sea salt)

- In a large size sauce pan, place all the ingredients and heat on medium, stirring and mixing, adjust the taste if you need more flavour with black pepper or chilli flakes.
- Simmer on low, once the pasta is cooked and drained add the pasta to the pan, and stir nicely. this is a wonderful base recipe to also add things like flaked tuna, grilled chicken chunks, grass fed meat balls, sautéed mushrooms, or grated pecorino.

2) Spaghetti delight

Ingredients

- Your choice of gluten free wholegrain spaghetti enough for 2 people
- 2 handfuls of cherry tomatoes cut in half
- Handful of pine nuts
- Sprinkle of sea salt and ground black pepper
- Grated Pecorino cheese to top off
- Olive oil

Instructions

- Boil water and cook spaghetti according to the instructions, add some olive oil and sea salt to the water
- Cut the tomatoes and set aside
- Heat the pine nuts on a pan until slightly golden brown
- In a medium size bowl add the pasta, and stir in the tomatoes, and pine nuts
- Top with ground black pepper and pecorino cheese

1) Casserole love

- 2 cups of whole grain gluten free penne or fusilli
- 1-2 small heads of chopped broccoli
- 1 cup of chopped and sautéed/ cooked/ sliced mushrooms

- Sea salt and black pepper
- 2 tsp of Minced garlic
- Drizzle of Olive oil for pasta
- Small amount of crumbled feta cheese

Instructions

- Boil water and cook pasta according to instructions
- Chop the broccoli and mushroom and set aside, next add some olive oil, garlic, sea salt and black pepper to a medium size pan and cook until slightly golden, add the broccoli first than add the mushrooms a couple of minutes later than set aside.
- Preheat your oven 200C,
- In a casserole style dish add the pasta, and stir in the veggies, next break up 1/4 to of the feta cheese, pop the dish in the oven to warm for a few minutes
- Sprinkle a little sea salt and ground black pepper before serving, give another stir
- Serve immediately

4) <u>Tacos</u>

Ingredients

- Your choice of organic lean protein, mushrooms, or vegan mince meat, make enough for 2 people.
- 1 cups of chopped iceberg lettuce
- 1 cup of chopped medium sized tomatoes
- 1 chopped deseeded red and green pepper
- 1 chopped and peeled avocado
- 1/2 cup of coconut yogurt
- Hot sauce
- Olive oil
- Generous pinch of chilli powder and paprika.
- 1 tbsp of coconut oil to cook your protein or plant protein
- Soft whole wheat/ gluten free wraps
- Grated vegan cheese or manchego cheese

Instructions

- Cook your type of protein adding the coconut oil in a pan until well done.
- Chop all the veggies, add to a big casserole style dish, toss, mix and add a drizzle of olive oil.
- Add a few drops of hot sauce to the coconut yogurt in a mini dipping bowl
- Warm the soft wraps, and arrange on your kitchen table, wraps, salad, and grated cheese and dips.
- Assemble yourself, and serve immediately.

5) <u>Asian fusion feast</u>

- 2 pieces of wild salmon or 2 portobello mushrooms
- 1 sliced courgette or a bunch of chopped kale
- 1 bunch of chopped broccoli
- 1 cup of chopped green beans
- 1 Tbsp of gluten free soya sauce
- Splash of fish sauce
- 2 tsp of minced garlic
- Little grated ginger
- Sprinkle of chilli flakes
- Drizzle of olive oil
- 1/2 lemon
- 1 tbsp of coconut oil

Instructions

- Preheat the oven to 180 degrees, and place the salmon fillets or portobello mushrooms in foil like a pouch, drizzle olive oil, and sprinkle a little sea salt and ground black pepper.
- In a big pan, heat coconut oil, add the soya sauce, fish sauce, very little grated ginger, garlic, and chill flakes
- Next add the chopped greens, and toss, stir and mix until all slightly golden brown, don't over cook, you want the heated and slightly crunchy.

- Serve in small bowls and add the salmon or mushrooms over the greens, and eat with chopsticks.
- Optional if you feel you want a little carb kick, use some rice noodles, or brown rice as a bottom base.

Sweet treats

Sweet potato shake muffins
Almond energy balls
Beauty bowl
Greek parfait
Vegan chocolate mousse

1) Sweet potato muffins

Ingredients

- 1 cup of cooked chopped sweet potato
- 1/2 cup of peanut butter or almond butter
- 1/4 cup of gluten free flour
- Scoop of a vegan plant protein powder
- Big drizzle of pure maple syrup
- 1 tsp of baking powder
- 1 Banana
- 3 Eggs
- Small handful of cacao nibs
- Sprinkle of sea salt

Instructions

- Preheat the oven to 200C, line 10-12 a muffin tin with the cupcake holders, turn to 180C before you pop in the oven.
- Combine all ingredients in one bowl, set aside
- Combine all wet ingredients and stir until smooth.
- Back for 15-18 minutes, until no muffin residue comes on a fork or tooth pick, keep checking them.
- Remove and chill, for a creamy touch

2) _Almond energy balls_

- 1 cup gluten free dry oats (I like 1/2 old fashioned oatmeal and 1/2 quick cooking)
- 1/4 cup smooth peanut butter or almond butter
- 1/4 cup pure maple syrup
- 1/2 cup cacao nibs
- small sprinkle of sea salt
- 1/2 teaspoon vanilla
- Sprinkle of chia or mixed seeds
- Sprinkle of maca or spirulina for mega energy boost

Instructions

- In a medium bowl, add all of the ingredients and stir to combine well. Chill in the fridge for at least half an hour.
- Use a spoon and scoop about a tablespoon of the cookie ball mixture into your hand. Roll into a ball. Repeat with remaining mixture.
- Store the balls covered in the fridge.

3) **Beauty bowl**

Serves 1 (just add more if there is more people)

- 1/2 cup of cooked gluten free oats
- 1/ 2 tbsp of coconut oil or ghee
- A little bit of almond milk to cook the oats in
- Small spoon of peanut butter or almond butter
- Sprinkle of your favourite superfoods powder like cacao, maca, spirulina
- Top off with half an avocado, small handful of blueberries, goji berries, chia seeds, shaved almonds, and deseeded pomegranates that you can easily buy at the supermarket ready to eat.
- Drizzle with maple syrup.

Instructions:

Make your gluten free oats in a small pan, heat the almond milk, add the coconut oil or ghee, than add the and cook according to instructions

- In a small bowl add your oats, then layer from left to right the toppings I have suggested.
- There are so many combos you can do with beauty bowls and make a great mid day lunch, mix it up with cooked quinoa, or brown rice as your base, get creative and switch up the toppings, with different superfoods, berries and nuts/ and seeds.

Beauty food feasting tip: Beauty bowls give you a mega dose of nourishment, energy and satisfaction in just one sitting, the best thing about them, is you can get creative in the kitchen and mix up your toppings, simply choose a gf whole grain base, and have fun with different fruits, flavours, superfoods, herbs and spices, depending if you fancy a bit of sweet or savoury, but make it plant based and pick 2-3 berries/. or fruits/ veg, a healthy fat, and 1-2 superfoods, voila and you have a instant healthy meal made in minutes.

<u>**Avo mousse**</u>

<u>**Ingredients**</u>

- 2 medium avocados
- 1/4 cup of coconut creme
- 1/2 cup of melted cacao nibs or buttons
- 2/3 cup of cacao powder
- 1 tsp of vanilla extract
- Dash of sea salt
- Handful of black berries for the topping

Instructions

- Add the avocados, maple syrup, coconut cream, melted cacao nibs, cacao powder, vanilla and salt to the food processor/ blend until smooth and thick.
- Transfer to 4 serving cute cups, top with blackberries, enjoy!

Greek parfait

Ingredients

- 1 1/2 cup of coconut yogurt
- Generous Drizzle of raw honey
- Ready to eat pomegranate seeds or passion fruit
- Sprinkle of Cacao nibs
- Top off with some crushed pistachios

Instructions

- Transfer and scoop some of the yogurt into 2 larger portion serving glasses or 4 small ones, than begin to layer each ingredient, yogurt, cacao nibs, fruit, honey, and repeat, 1 -2 more times, lastly drizzle with a little raw honey, and sprinkle of pistachios
- Place to chill in the fridge for at least 30 minutes to help it set. Enjoy

Wake up liquid elixir

Make first thing in the morning upon awakening and sip on a empty stomach, if you are short for time, a fab way to grab and go is make a batch for the weekdays on a Sunday night, so it's ready to drink, simply multiply the recipe by 5 and store in a mason jar.

Ingredients

- 1-2 juice of lemons
- Big pinch of turmeric powder

- Big pinch of ground pepper
- Drizzle of raw honey or maple syrup
- Small cup of warm or room temperature filtered water
- Optional pinch of cayenne pepper and a little grated ginger
- For extra cleansing and alkalising properties, I love steeping 1-2 bags of detox tea (there are many on the market), then adding the elixir blend to it, literally you feel your system getting a good clean up first thing in the morning

Beauty boosting smoothies

Coco berry

- 1 large handful of blueberries
- 1 large handful of raspberries
- 1 handfuls of spinach
- 1 cup of coconut water
- 1/2 avocado
- 1 scoop a plant based shake
- 1-2 other types of superfoods

Add all ingredients to a blender, blend until smooth, drink immediately.

Creamy Kale berry Banana

- 1 large handful of blueberries
- 1 large handful of blackberries
- 2 large handfuls of kale
- 1 cup of almond milk
- 1/2 banana
- 1 scoop of a plant based vega shake
- 1–2 superfoods

Add all ingredients to a blender, blend until smooth, drink immediately.

Cleansing Cucumber Berry

- 1 large handful of strawberries
- 1 large handful of blueberries
- 2 large handfuls of rocket
- 1 cucumber
- 1 cup of aloe vera juice

Add all ingredients to a blender, blend until smooth, drink immediately.

Berry butter

- 1 large handful of blueberries
- 1 handful of strawberries
- 1 handfuls of leafy greens
- 1 spoonful of peanut butter
- 1 cup of almond milk
- 1/2 banana
- 1 scoop of plant based powder
- 1–2 superfoods of your choosing

Add all ingredients to a blender, blend until smooth, drink immediately.

Mango berry Hemp shake

- 1 handful of chopped mangos
- 1 handful of blueberries
- 1 handful of strawberries
- 1 cup of hemp milk
- 1 handfuls of leafy greens
- 1 cup of mineral water
- 1 scoop of Vega shake
- 1–2 superfoods

Add all ingredients to a blender, blend until smooth, drink immediately.

Sexy Salad Dressings

In a food processor blend one of the following for a delicious and nutritious finish to your salad

1) **Strawberry Basil:** 2 Tbsp of Olive oil, 1 Tbsp of Balsamic Vinegar, 2 Tsp of Raw honey, 1 Cup of strawberries, 1/8 of cup of chopped basil.

2) **Pomegranate Cilantro:** 2 Tbsp of Olive oil, 1 Tbsp of White wine vinegar, 1 cup of deseeded pomegranates, 1 Tbsp of raw honey, 1/8 of a cup of chopped cilantro

3) **Lemon and Ginger:** 2 Tbsp of Olive oil. 2 juice of lemons. 2 Tbsp of Ginger grated. 1 Tsp of Turmeric. 2 Tbsp of raw honey

4) **Orange and Cayenne Pepper:** 2 Tbsp of Olive oil, 1 tsp of Tamari sauce, 2 juice of Oranges. pinch of cayenne pepper, 2 Tbsp of maple syrup

5) **Blueberry Basil:** 2 Tbsp of Olive oil, 1 Tbsp of Apple cider vinegar, 1/2 cup of blueberries. 1/8 cup of basil. 1 Tbsp of raw honey. 1 Tsp of minced garlic

6) **Sweet Goji & Cilantro:** 2 Tbsp of Avocado oil. 1/3 cup of goji berries, 1/2 Tsp of Balsamic vinegar, 1/2 cup of cilantro, 2 tbsp of raw honey

AUTHOR BIO

Ashley Siedentopf is a Certified Nutritionist and Integrative Nutrition Health Coach, author and online health talk host. She is passionate about life, wellness, wine, fashion, yoga, skincare, spiritulatiy, travel, real estate and organic healthy living. She resides in London, with her husband, daughter, and pug.

Printed in the United States
By Bookmasters